MOSBY'S
Fluids & Electrolytes
Memory
NoteCards
Visual, Mnemonic, and Memory Aids for Nurses

JoAnn Zerwekh, EdD, RN
President/CEO
Nursing Education Consultants
Chandler, Arizona
Nursing Faculty–Online Campus
Upper Iowa University
Mesa, Arizona

CJ Miller, BSN, RN
Illustrator
Cedar Rapids, Iowa

T0200386

ELSEVIER

MOSBY
ELSEVIER
3251 Riverport Lane
St. Louis, MO 63043

MOSBY'S FLUIDS & ELECTROLYTES
MEMORY NOTECARDS: VISUAL, MNEMONIC,
AND MEMORY AIDS FOR NURSES   ISBN-13: 978-0-323-83225-0

Notice

Nursing is an ever-changing field. Standard safety precautions must be followed, but as new research and clinical experience broaden our knowledge, changes in treatment and drug therapy may become necessary or appropriate. Readers are advised to check the most current product information provided by the manufacturer of each drug to be administered to verify the recommended dose, the method and duration of administration, and contraindications. It is the responsibility of the licensed prescriber, relying on experience and knowledge of the patient, to determine dosages and the best treatment for each individual patient. Neither the publisher nor the editor assumes any liability for any injury and/or damage to persons or property arising from this publication.

International Standard Book Number: 978-0-323-83225-0
Content Strategist: Heather Bays-Petrovic
Sr Content Development Manager: Somodatta Roy Choudhury
Publishing Services Manager: Deepthi Unni
Project Manager: Aparna Venkatachalam
Designer: Brian Salisbury
Illustration Buyer: Nijantha Priyadharshini

Printed in India

Last digit is the print number: 9   8   7   6   5   4   3   2   1

FLUIDS & ELECTROLYTES, 1

ACID-BASE BALANCE, 83

FINALLY, FLUIDS & ELECTROLYTES AND ACID-BASE BALANCE MADE CLEAR!

Use Your New Notecards As A:

- Pocket reference for clinicals
- Companion study guide for pharmacology texts
- Quick review for exams
- Patient teaching aid
- Resource for writing nursing care plans

Changes to this edition include the integration of NCSBN's Clinical Judgment Measurement Model (NCJMM):

- The nurse identifies patient needs and makes a clinical decision about what to do, which involves clinical judgment.
- The following are the six cognitive skills in the NCJMM that are used to make sound clinical judgments related to patient care: recognize cues, analyze cues, prioritize hypotheses, generate solutions, take action, evaluate outcomes. For the purposes of understanding fluid and electrolytes, acid-base balance, and intravenous therapy, only 3 of these cognitive skills have been identified in this handy flip-card reference.
- Signs and symptoms, abnormal findings, and diagnostic tests have been included in a newly titled section – **Assessment: Recognize Cues.**
- Medical management, which includes having knowledge about medications and treatments that are incorporated into a plan of care has been renamed – **Medical Management: Generate Solutions.**
- Nursing management, which includes nursing interventions has been renamed – **Nursing Management: Take Action.**

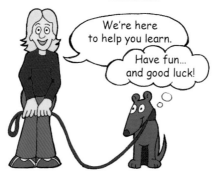

HOMEOSTASIS:
A QUESTION OF BALANCE

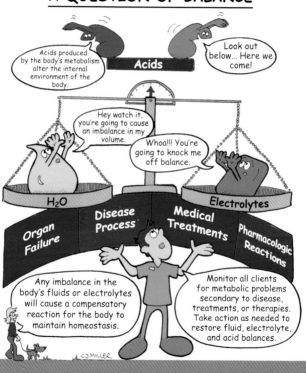

What You Need to Know
Homeostasis

SIGNIFICANCE OF HOMEOSTASIS

Homeostasis is considered the steady state of the body by which the internal systems of the body maintain a balance, despite external conditions. This natural state of equilibrium is maintained by adaptive responses that promote healthy functioning of the body.

EXAMPLES OF HOMEOSTASIS

Homeostasis occurs when the body regulates temperature in an effort to maintain an internal temperature of approximately 98.6° Fahrenheit (F) or 37° Celsius (C). Sweating cools the body on a hot day, and shivering produces heat on a cold day, both of which are accomplished primarily through the skin. These compensatory mechanisms maintain a steady state in the body related to temperature. Other examples of homeostasis are the regulation of the amounts of water and minerals in the body by the kidneys (osmoregulation), the excretion of metabolic waste by the excretory organs such as the kidneys, the regulation of pH levels in the blood and lungs with the exchange of oxygen and carbon dioxide, and the regulation of blood glucose levels by the liver and insulin secreted by the pancreas.

HOMEOSTASIS AND ELECTROLYTE BALANCE

For the body to maintain a state of equilibrium, the composition and volume of body fluids need to be kept within a narrow range that is considered normal. The body's normal metabolism creates acids as end-products. These acids (carbonic acids) can alter the normal internal balance.

STRESS

Stress disturbs homeostasis and causes the body to try to adapt to the stressor. Stress stimulates the hypothalamic-pituitary-adrenal (HPA) axis for the maintenance of homeostasis in response to challenges. Examples of physical stress include hypoglycemia, trauma, exposure to extreme temperatures, infections, or heavy exercise. Examples of psychologic stress include acute anxiety, chronic anxiety, or anticipation of stressful situations.

Important nursing implications	Serious/life-threatening implications
Most frequent side effects	Patient teaching

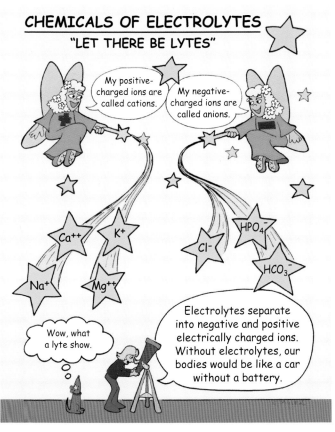

=========== **What You Need to Know** ===========
Electrolyte Overview

SIGNIFICANCE OF ELECTROLYTES

Electrolytes are substances found in the intracellular fluid (ICF) and extracellular fluid (ECF) whose molecules split into ions when placed in water. The major electrolytes found in the body are potassium, sodium, calcium, chloride, phosphorus, and magnesium. Electrolytes are distinguished by their electrical charge as either positive or negative. Electrolytes that have a positive charge are known as *cations*. Electrolytes that have a negative charge are known as *anions*. Examples of cations are potassium, sodium, magnesium, and calcium. Examples of anions are bicarbonate, chloride, and phosphate. Without electrolytes, the body cannot maintain homeostasis.

SOURCES OF ELECTROLYTES

Electrolytes can be found in the following foods:
- Fruits, vegetables, and grains
- Red meat, poultry, and fish
- Fluids
- Supplements

CONTROL OF ELECTROLYTES

Electrolytes are regulated in the body by their degree of concentration. Diffusion, active transport, and osmosis are mechanisms that maintain electrolyte balance in the body.

Diffusion is a process that moves molecules from an area of higher concentration to an area of lower concentration. No energy is required.

Active transport occurs when molecules move across the concentration gradient. The sodium-potassium pump is an example of active transport. Sodium moves out of the cell as potassium moves into the cell to maintain a steady concentration balance. Adenosine triphosphate (ATP) is the energy required for this process and is made in the cell mitochondria.

Osmosis is the process during which water moves down a concentration gradient from an area that contains more water (a dilute area) to an area that has less water (high solute concentration). *The concentration of the solution determines the strength of the osmotic pull. The higher the concentration, the greater a solution's pull, or* **osmotic pressure.**

FUNCTIONS OF ELECTROLYTES

- Maintain homeostasis
- Regulate fluid balance
- Maintain acid-base balance

FLUID BALANCE: A MATTER FOR THE BRAIN AND KIDNEYS

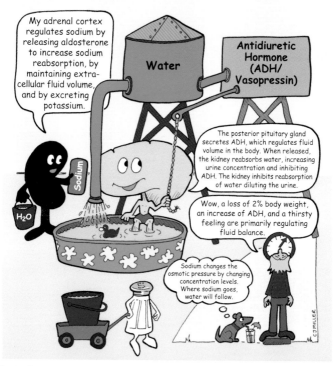

What You Need to Know
Overview of Fluid Balance

SIGNIFICANCE OF FLUID BALANCE

The term *fluid balance* defines the body's state in which a required amount of water is present and is distributed among the various body fluid compartments (ICF and ECF). Essentially, the body is in fluid balance when water intake equals water loss. This state of fluid balance is inseparable from electrolyte balance. When the intake of water is greater than the loss of water, or vice versa, then fluid imbalance results. Fluid balance is a necessary component in maintaining homeostasis.

SOURCES OF FLUIDS

- Water and any other liquid that can be ingested
- Intravenous (IV) fluids
- Fruits and vegetables

CONTROL OF FLUIDS

Fluid balance is regulated in the body by the body's own thirst mechanism, as well as by the hypothalamus, the pituitary and adrenal glands, the kidneys, and the gastrointestinal (GI) system. Insensible water loss or fluid that cannot be measured accounts for approximately 500 to 1000 mL of fluid loss in the adult per day.

Thirst mechanism is initiated when a person's body fluid decreases. Osmo-receptors in the hypothalamus initiate a stimulus that senses a need for fluids.

The hypothalamus makes antidiuretic hormone (ADH), and the posterior pituitary gland stores the ADH until the hypothalamus initiates a signal to the pituitary gland, causing ADH to be released. Once ADH is released in the body, the distal tubules of the kidneys respond by reabsorbing water. After a person drinks a glass of water, ADH prevents it from becoming excreted.

The adrenal cortex secretes aldosterone (mineralocorticoid), which has properties of sodium reabsorption and potassium excretion. Important to remember, water follows salt. As sodium is reabsorbed, water follows because of an osmotic change.

The kidneys regulate fluid balance by adjusting the amount of urine volume that is excreted. An adult excretes 1.5 L of urine per day on average or a minimum of 30 mL/hr (0.5 to 1.5mL/kg/hr). For children, the expected urine output is 1 mL/kg/hr.

The GI tract is responsible for absorbing water intake. A small amount of fluid is lost in feces. However, diarrhea and vomiting can cause major fluid volume deficits, because 3 to 6 L of fluid is secreted and reabsorbed into the GI tract daily.

THE BODY'S WATER: KEEPING IT WHERE YOU NEED IT

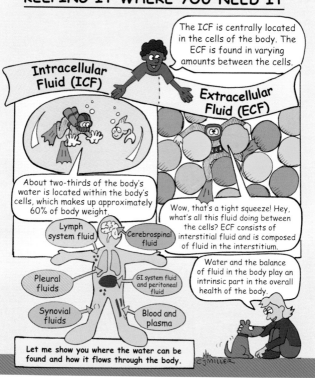

=== **What You Need to Know** ===
The Body's Water

SIGNIFICANCE OF WATER

Water makes up approximately 60% of total body weight and moves freely among body compartments and is distributed by osmotic and hydrostatic forces. Approximately two-thirds of body water is ICF and one-third is ECF. The ECF has two main compartments: (1) *interstitial fluid,* which is fluid in the space between the cells and lymph glands, and (2) *intravascular fluid,* which is fluid found in blood plasma. Small amounts of fluid are contained in the cerebrospinal fluid and in the GI tract, as well as in pleural, synovial, and peritoneal fluid, which is often called *transcellular fluid.* Under normal conditions, water loss equals water gain and a body's water volume remains constant.

AGE CONSIDERATIONS OF WATER BALANCE

Total body water can be significantly lower in obese individuals and in the older adult. The older adult has increased body fat and decreased muscle and a reduced ability to regulate sodium and water balance. Fever and dehydration can lead to significant fluid balance problems for the older adult. Infants have more body water, approximately 75% to 80% of body weight, because they have less fat. Infants are more susceptible to changes in body water because of their high metabolic rate and their greater body surface area in proportion to body size. Loss of fluids from diarrhea can have significant fluid balance effects on the infant.

FUNCTIONS OF BODY WATER

- Transports nutrients, electrolytes, and oxygen to cells
- Carries water products away from cells
- Regulates body temperature
- Lubricates joints and mucous membranes
- Medium for chemical reactions in the body
- Aids in food digestion

Important nursing implications	Serious/life-threatening implications
Most frequent side effects	Patient teaching

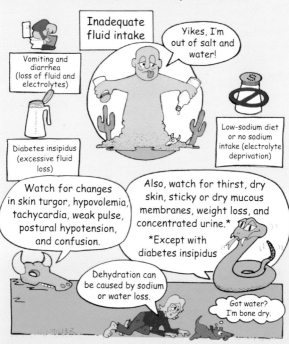

=== **What You Need to Know** ===
Dehydration and Fluid Volume Deficit

GENERAL

Dehydration describes a significant decrease in fluid intake and/or a loss of body fluid without replacement. A fluid volume deficit occurs with the loss of body fluids (e.g., diarrhea, vomiting, hemorrhage, fistula drainage, polyuria) or can be caused by an inadequate intake of fluids or a plasma-to-interstitial fluid shift. The causes of a fluid volume deficit include the following:

- Insensible water loss or perspiration (e.g., high fever, heatstroke)
- Diabetes insipidus, osmotic diuresis, or hemorrhage
- GI losses—vomiting, suction, diarrhea, and fistula drainage
- Overuse of diuretic agents and inadequate fluid intake
- Third-spacing of fluids—burns and intestinal obstruction

ASSESSMENT: RECOGNIZE CUES

Moderate signs and symptoms of dehydration and fluid volume deficit include:

- Flushed dry skin
- Dry mucous membranes, tenting (skin turgor), and decreased urine output
- Urine characteristics: increased specific gravity (color may be dark yellow to amber)
- Thirst and weight loss
- Restlessness and lethargy
  Severe signs and symptoms of dehydration and fluid volume deficit include:
- Dry, cracked tongue and soft, sunken eyeballs
- Thready pulse, tachycardia, and decreased central venous pressure (CVP)
- Postural hypotension and rapid respiratory rate
- Lethargy progressing to coma
- Absence of tearing or sweating
- Oliguric or very concentrated urine
- Hemoconcentration—increased hematocrit (Hct), blood urea nitrogen (BUN), and electrolytes; hemoconcentration does not occur when dehydration is caused by hemorrhage

DIAGNOSTIC FINDINGS

- Urine specific gravity >1.020
- Elevated hemoglobin (Hgb) and Hct levels
- Elevated potassium levels

NURSING MANAGEMENT OF FLUID VOLUME DEFICIT

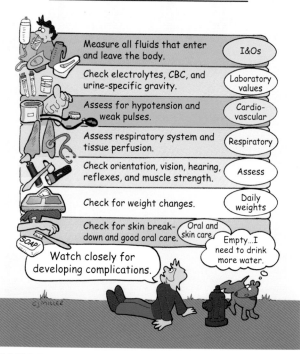

Measure all fluids that enter and leave the body.	I&Os
Check electrolytes, CBC, and urine-specific gravity.	Laboratory values
Assess for hypotension and weak pulses.	Cardio-vascular
Assess respiratory system and tissue perfusion.	Respiratory
Check orientation, vision, hearing, reflexes, and muscle strength.	Assess
Check for weight changes.	Daily weights
Check for skin break-down and good oral care.	Oral and skin care

Empty...I need to drink more water.

Watch closely for developing complications.

Fluids & Electrolytes

===== **What You Need to Know** =====
Management of Fluid Volume Deficit

MEDICAL MANAGEMENT: GENERATE SOLUTIONS

- Restore fluid loss, which is the goal of treatment.
- Determine the amount of IV fluid replacement, which will depend on the type and severity of fluid loss.
- Provide isotonic solutions (0.9%) or balanced IV solutions (lactated Ringer's solution), which are usually used in the initial treatment.

NURSING MANAGEMENT: TAKE ACTION

- Identify clients at increased risk for fluid volume deficit.
- Monitor vital signs and assess for postural hypotension.
- Measure total intake and output (I&O) and document it.
- Obtain accurate daily weights.
- Evaluate urinary output and specific gravity.
- Monitor serum laboratory values for concentrations of Hct, BUN, and sodium.
- Monitor Hgb and Hct (H&H) levels.
- Assess client's level of consciousness.
- Evaluate the client's response to fluid replacement (urine output and weight).
- Encourage the client to increase oral intake before performing any strenuous activity.
- Teach the client the importance of consuming at least 64 oz of water daily to prevent dehydration.
  Additional nursing management considerations include the following:
- Skin turgor is a poor indication of hydration status in the older adult.
- Hypovolemic shock is a serious complication associated with fluid volume deficit, which is the result of inadequate blood volume to maintain normal circulation.
- Change in mentation may occur in severe fluid volume deficits.

Important nursing implications	Serious/life-threatening implications
Most frequent side effects	Patient teaching

FLUID VOLUME EXCESS

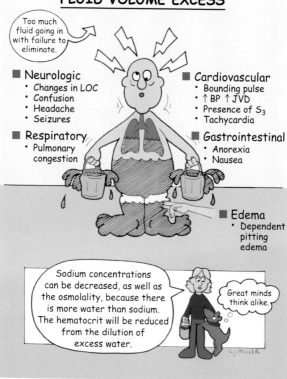

Too much fluid going in with failure to eliminate.

- **Neurologic**
  - Changes in LOC
  - Confusion
  - Headache
  - Seizures

- **Respiratory**
  - Pulmonary congestion

- **Cardiovascular**
  - Bounding pulse
  - ↑ BP ↑ JVD
  - Presence of S_3
  - Tachycardia

- **Gastrointestinal**
  - Anorexia
  - Nausea

- **Edema**
  - Dependent pitting edema

Sodium concentrations can be decreased, as well as the osmolality, because there is more water than sodium. The hematocrit will be reduced from the dilution of excess water.

Great minds think alike.

Fluid Volume Excess

GENERAL

When the body (i.e., kidneys, liver, heart) is functioning normally, it is difficult for the body to have an excess of fluids. When excess water is retained, it causes a dilution of the ECF, and water moves into the ICF. Fluid volume excess is caused by excessive intake of fluids (e.g., rapid infusion of IV fluids, excessive isotonic or hypotonic IV fluids), retention of fluids, kidney failure, Cushing syndrome, long-term use of corticosteroids, syndrome of inappropriate antidiuretic hormone (SIADH) secretion, primary polydipsia, or an interstitial-to-plasma fluid shift. Edema may exist in fluid volume excess, but edema and fluid volume excess are not the same.

Fluid volume excess is also called *water intoxication* in individuals who engage in compulsive water drinking.

ASSESSMENT: RECOGNIZE CUES

- Edema—peripheral pitting; skin pale and cool to touch
- Jugular vein distention (JVD)
- Respiratory difficulty, shortness of breath (SOB), moist breath sounds, and coughing
- Weight gain
- Mental confusion and lethargy
- Visual disturbances
- Muscle cramping, paresthesias, and muscle weakness
- Nausea, increased GI motility
- Enlarged liver (hepatomegaly)
- Cerebral edema

DIAGNOSTIC FINDINGS

- Hyponatremia, dilutional (serum sodium level <135 mEq/L)
- Decreased BUN
- Decreased Hgb &Hct levels
- Decreased serum protein
- Decreased serum and urine osmolarity

Important nursing implications	Serious/life-threatening implications
Most frequent side effects	Patient teaching

NURSING MANAGEMENT OF FLUID VOLUME EXCESS

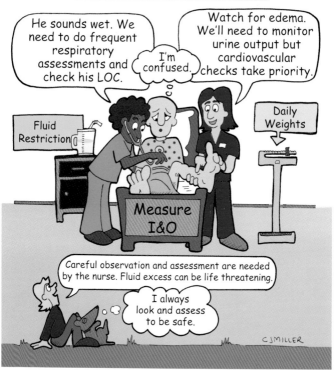

What You Need to Know
Management of Fluid Volume Excess

MEDICAL MANAGEMENT: GENERATE SOLUTIONS

- Decrease the amount of fluid in the cells, which is the goal of treatment.
- Assess and, if needed, administer hypertonic IV solution.
- Administer diuretics to increase kidney excretion of water and sodium. Their action works by reversing the osmotic gradient and pulling water out of the cell.

NURSING MANAGEMENT: TAKE ACTION

- Monitor the client for a change in mentation.
  - Change in mentation is an early sign of cerebral edema.
- Assess the client q2h to monitor for pulmonary edema, which may occur quickly and lead to death.
- Monitor daily weight.
- Monitor I&O.
- Decrease the intake of water and sodium.
- Elevate the head of the bed.
- Encourage mobility.
- Monitor electrolytes—especially potassium and sodium.
- Assess the client's history of conditions that may cause fluid retention: heart failure, kidney failure, Cushing syndrome, prolonged use of corticosteroids, SIADH, or high salt intake.
- Teach the client to limit intake of oral fluids.
- Inform the client of the early signs and symptoms associated with water retention.
- Rapid weight gain is the best indication of fluid retention and overload (1 L of fluid equals 2.2 kg, or 1 pound).

Important nursing implications   Serious/life-threatening implications

Most frequent side effects   Patient teaching

HEATSTROKE

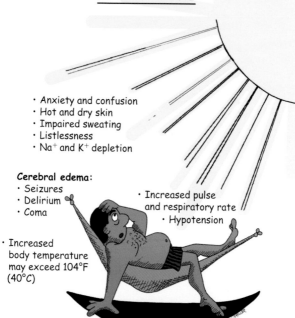

- Anxiety and confusion
- Hot and dry skin
- Impaired sweating
- Listlessness
- Na^+ and K^+ depletion

Cerebral edema:
- Seizures
- Delirium
- Coma

- Increased pulse and respiratory rate
- Hypotension

- Increased body temperature may exceed 104°F (40°C)

Management—Cooling, rest, and fluid & electrolyte support

Fluids & Electrolytes

=== **What You Need to Know** ===
Management of Heatstroke

MEDICAL MANAGEMENT: GENERATE SOLUTIONS

- Heatstroke is a medical emergency—body temperature may exceed 104°F (40°C).
- Administer a high concentration of oxygen therapy.
- Provide IV of normal saline; avoid hypotonic fluids. Do not use lactated Ringer's solution because the liver cannot metabolize the lactate, which can worsen lactic acidosis.
- Insert a urinary catheter.
- Place a continuous core temperature monitoring device to prevent hypothermia during aggressive cooling treatment. Do not rely on oral temperature—a rectal temperature is always preferred.
- Administer midazolam or propofol if shivering occurs. Patient is at risk for delirium with midazolam and hypotension with propofol.
- Give benzodiazepines for seizures caused by elevated temperatures.
- Aspirin and other antipyretics are contraindicated.

NURSING MANAGEMENT: TAKE ACTION

- In the prehospital setting, rapid cooling is the first priority.
  - Remove the client's clothing.
  - Immerse the client in cold water.
  - Wet the body with tepid water, and then fan to promote cooling.
- Provide aggressive intervention to cool the client.
  - Provide cooling blankets and ice packs to the axilla, groin, neck, and head.
  - Monitor procedures for internal cooling methods of iced gastric and bladder lavage and, in severe cases, iced peritoneal lavage.
  - Begin slow cooling when the core body temperature is reduced to 102° F.
- Monitor vital signs, urine output, and specific gravity.
- Monitor for complications such as multiple-organ dysfunction syndrome (MODS), kidney impairment, electrolyte and acid-base problems, pulmonary edema, and cerebral edema.
- Instruct the client to avoid situations that may precipitate heatstroke (e.g., strenuous activity in hot weather; too heavy clothing for climate; chronic exposure to hot, humid environments).
- Teach groups at risk for heatstroke (ill and older adults) to avoid situations that may lead to heatstroke.

SODIUM

"IT'S OUTSIDE THE CELL IN THE EXTRACELLULAR FLUID"

Sodium is 90% of the ECF cations, and that makes it positive! Sodium always hangs out with its negative anion friends—chloride and bicarbonate.

Interstitial sodium surrounds cells of the body.

Circulatory or intravascular fluid or plasma sodium throughout the body.

Transcellular fluid is found in joint body and organ spaces.

Sodium also works with K^+ and Ca^{++} to conduct nerve impulses and regulate acid-base balance. It is also involved with cellular chemical reactions.

Don't forget it helps with membrane transport.

Fluids & Electrolytes

What You Need to Know
Sodium

SIGNIFICANCE OF SODIUM

Sodium is the major cation found in the ECF, and its role is to maintain fluid volume in the body. The normal laboratory values of sodium are 135 to 145 mEq/L. Changes in sodium levels significantly change fluid volume and the distribution of other electrolytes.

SOURCES OF SODIUM

- Table salt, seasonings, and spices
- Processed and smoked foods
- Hot dogs, cold cuts, beef jerky, and canned soup
- Saltine crackers, pretzels, and potato chips
- Canned soda beverages
- Pickles and other pickled foods
- Sardines and herring
- Potatoes and other white vegetables

CONTROL OF SODIUM

Sodium is controlled by several mechanisms in the body:
- Osmoreceptors send a message to the brain when too much sodium is in the ECF, and this message initiates the thirst mechanism, which causes the person to drink a glass of water to quench their thirst.
- The hypothalamus stimulates the pituitary gland to release ADH. ADH helps retain body fluids.
- The kidneys will now hold onto this extra fluid in the body to decrease the serum osmolality of the sodium (sodium will follow the water).
- Aldosterone promotes sodium reabsorption from the distal renal tubules.

FUNCTIONS OF SODIUM

- Regulates osmolality
- Helps maintain blood pressure (BP) by balancing the volume of water in the body
- Works with other electrolytes to promote the transmission of nerve impulses to muscles and tissues
- Involved with muscle contractility
- Helps maintain acid-base balance

HYPERNATREMIA

Hello brain...this is the hypothalamus. Say, we've got a problem. Sodium and osmolality are up...my guy here is real thirsty.

Brain here...thanks for the info. I'll pass it on to the pituitary gland.

Pituitary gland here...I'm releasing the antidiuretic hormone (ADH).

Hypernatremia: Sodium >145 mEq/L

Hyponatremia: Sodium <135 mEq/L

I'm so thirsty!

Kidney here... I'm cutting back on urine output to increase dilution of sodium and osmolality.

Hypernatremia (fluid volume deficit)—watch for signs of thirst, fever, dry mucous membranes, hypotension, tachycardia, low jugular venous pressure, and restlessness.

That's it...no more chips and dip!

Chips

Fluids & Electrolytes

What You Need to Know
Hypernatremia

GENERAL

When serum sodium levels are >145 mEq/L, hypernatremia is the resulting condition. Hypernatremia may develop as a result of one of several problems:

- Dehydration due to volume deficit, which causes an increase in the concentration of the sodium in the serum
- Excessive sodium intake
- Interruption of the body's regulatory mechanism for sodium

Hypernatremia can occur from several factors: (1) eating a high-sodium meal or not drinking enough fluids, which leads to fluid volume deficit; (2) excessive water loss (e.g., high fever, heatstroke, diarrhea); or (3) administering IV fluids that are considered hypertonic (e.g., hypertonic sodium chloride [NaCl], excessive isotonic NaCl, sodium bicarbonate).

Other disease processes that can interrupt the body's sodium regulatory mechanism include diabetes insipidus, kidney failure, primary hyperaldosteronism, Cushing syndrome, and uncontrolled diabetes mellitus.

Medications that promote osmotic diuresis (mannitol) may also cause hypernatremia, a condition in which fluid is lost and sodium is concentrated.

ASSESSMENT: RECOGNIZE CUES

- Irritability, restlessness, confusion, and twitching
- Increased thirst and dry mucous membranes
- Decreased urinary output
- Dyspnea or pulmonary edema from sodium gain
- Flushed skin
- Orthostatic hypotension (fluid loss)

DIAGNOSTIC FINDINGS

- Serum sodium >145 mEq/L
- Serum osmolality >300 mOsm/kg
- Specific gravity >1.030

HEMODYNAMIC MEASUREMENTS

- Sodium excess—elevated CVP and pulmonary artery pressure (PAP)
- Water loss—decreased CVP and PAP

HYPERNATREMIA
"YOU ARE FRIED"

F Fever (low grade), flushed skin

R Restless (irritable)

I Increased fluid retention and ↑ BP

E Edema (peripheral and pitting)

D Decreased urine output, dry mouth

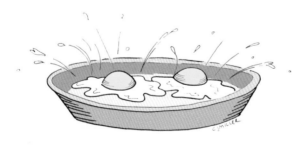

What You Need to Know
Hypernatremia—FRIED

GENERAL

The acronym FRIED is a mnemonic to help you remember the signs and symptoms of hypernatremia with normal or increased ECF volume. Think of the body heat of a fever and the heat of a frying pan—the visual image will help you associate the two.

When serum sodium levels are >145 mEq/L, hypernatremia is the resulting condition. It most often occurs when water intake decreases, leading to an increased sodium concentration.

ASSESSMENT: RECOGNIZE CUES

The first five signs and symptoms of hypernatremia with normal or increased ECF volume make up the acronym FRIED:
- **F**ever (low grade) and flushed skin
- **R**estlessness, irritability, and confusion
- **I**ncreased fluid retention and increased BP
- **E**dema (peripheral and pitting)
- **D**ecreased urinary output, dry mouth, and increased thirst
- Twitching
- Dyspnea
- Elevated CVP and PAP
- Pulmonary edema, seizures, and coma

NURSING MANAGEMENT: TAKE ACTION

- Monitor that the serum sodium level so that it does not decrease by more than 8 to 15 mEq/L in an 8-hour period.
- Quickly reducing sodium levels can cause a rapid shift of water back into the cells causing cerebral edema and neurologic complications.
  - This risk is greatest if hypernatremia developed over several days or longer.

Important nursing implications	Serious/life-threatening implications
Most frequent side effects	Patient teaching

24

HYPERNATREMIA

"THE MODEL"
(Causes of ↑ serum sodium)

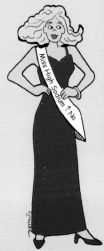

M Medications, meals
(too much sodium intake)

O Osmotic diuretics

D Diabetes insipidus

E Excessive H_2O loss

L Low H_2O intake

What You Need to Know
Hypernatremia—MODEL

GENERAL

The acronym MODEL emphasizes **M**edication and meals, **O**smotic diuretic agents, **D**iabetes insipidus, **E**xcessive water loss, and **L**ow water intake.

The trick is to mentally attach the picture and acronym to the symptoms to enhance memory recall.

When serum sodium levels are >145 mEq/L, hypernatremia is the resulting condition.

Hypernatremia can be caused by several factors: (1) eating a high-sodium meal; (2) not drinking enough fluids, leading to dehydration; or (3) administering IV fluids that are considered hypertonic (hypertonic NaCl, excessive isotonic NaCl, or sodium bicarbonate).

Some other disease processes that can cause hypernatremia are diabetes insipidus, kidney failure, primary hyperaldosteronism, Cushing syndrome, long-term use of corticosteroids, and uncontrolled diabetes mellitus.

Medications that promote osmotic diuresis (mannitol) may also cause hypernatremia.

CAUSES OF HYPERNATREMIA: ANALYZE CUES

- **M**edications and meals (too much salt intake)
- **O**smotic diuretic agents (mannitol)
- **D**iabetes insipidus
- **E**xcessive water loss
- **L**ow water intake

Important nursing implications	Serious/life-threatening implications
Most frequent side effects	Patient teaching

NURSING MANAGEMENT OF HYPERNATREMIA

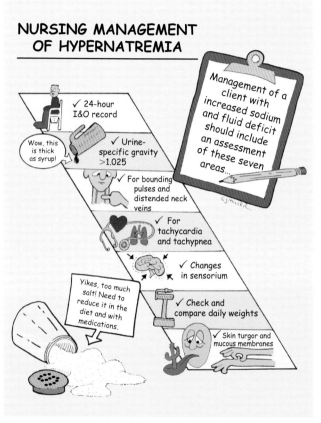

What You Need to Know
Management of Hypernatremia

GENERAL

The treatment for hypernatremia depends on the cause—either water lost or sodium gained. Corrections should be provided slowly to avoid a shift of water into the cerebral cells leading to cerebral edema.

MEDICAL MANAGEMENT: GENERATE SOLUTIONS

- Administer diuretic therapy, which promotes the excretion of sodium.
  - Furosemide or bumetanide may be given.
  - Assess hourly for indications of excessive losses of fluid, sodium, and potassium following drug therapy.
- Provide hydration therapy.
- Administer isotonic saline (0.9%) or dextrose 5% in 0.45% NaCl. Although the dextrose 5% in 0.45% NaCl is hypertonic in the IV bag, once it is infused, the glucose is rapidly metabolized making the infused fluid hypotonic.
- Treat the underlying cause.
  - If a too rapid infusion of hypertonic solution is a contributing cause, the rate should be decreased.
  - The client is questioned about their daily diet (high sodium–containing foods may be a contributing cause).
- Provide fluids, if the client is dehydrated.

NURSING MANAGEMENT: TAKE ACTION

- Monitor vital signs.
  - Tachycardia
  - Increased BP with fluid overload and decreased BP with fluid deficit
  - Increased temperature >101°F (38°C)
- Measure I&O.
- Obtain daily weight (before breakfast or at the same time each day).
  - Make sure the client is wearing the same type of clothes from the previous day and uses the same scale.
  - Inform the client that a weight gain of 2 lb or more in a 4-day period should be reported to the healthcare provider immediately.
  - A loss of 4.4 lb is approximately a loss of 2 L of fluid.
- Assess for edema in the peripheral extremities, sacrum, and face.
- Monitor the client for risk of seizures.

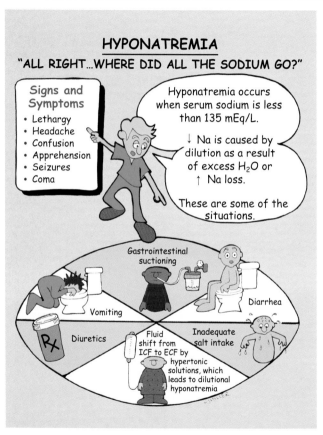

HYPONATREMIA
"ALL RIGHT...WHERE DID ALL THE SODIUM GO?"

Signs and Symptoms
- Lethargy
- Headache
- Confusion
- Apprehension
- Seizures
- Coma

Hyponatremia occurs when serum sodium is less than 135 mEq/L.

↓ Na is caused by dilution as a result of excess H_2O or ↑ Na loss.

These are some of the situations.

Gastrointestinal suctioning

Diarrhea

Vomiting

Inadequate salt intake

Diuretics

Fluid shift from ICF to ECF by hypertonic solutions, which leads to dilutional hyponatremia

Fluids & Electrolytes

What You Need to Know
Hyponatremia

GENERAL

When serum sodium concentration in the body decreases, the condition is known as *hyponatremia.* Hyponatremia may be caused by excessive dilution of the sodium by fluid volume excess or by an increase in sodium loss from the body. Hyponatremia is defined a serum sodium level of <135 mEq/L. With severe hyponatremia, an ICF shift may occur that will result in cerebral edema.

The following may cause hyponatremia:
- IV fluid overload with an inappropriate use of sodium-free or hypotonic IV fluids (fluid gain) (the most common cause)
- Fluid overload after drinking water (fluid gain)
- Dilutional states (e.g., hyperglycemia, SIADH, heart failure) (fluid gain)
- Aggressive diuretic therapy (sodium loss)
- GI drainage, diarrhea, vomiting, and fistulas (sodium loss)
- Excessive sweating (sodium loss)

ASSESSMENT: RECOGNIZE CUES

Sodium Loss
- Irritability, apprehension, and confusion
- Postural hypotension; tachycardia; and rapid and weak, thready pulse
- Decreased CVP and decreased jugular vein filling
- Weight loss and dry mucous membranes
- Tremors, seizures, and coma
- <125 mEq/L (neurologic signs are assessed for cerebral edema)

Fluid Gain
- Headache, apathy, and confusion
- Weight gain, increased BP, and elevated CVP
- Hallmark signs: nausea, vomiting, anorexia, lethargy, and weakness
- When muscle weakness is present, immediately check respiratory status because ventilation depends on adequate strength of respiratory muscles.
- Increased urinary output
- Cerebral edema

DIAGNOSTIC FINDINGS
- Serum sodium <135 mEq/L
- Urine specific gravity <1.010
- Critical level serum sodium <110 mEq/L

Hyponatremia
" LOW SALT"

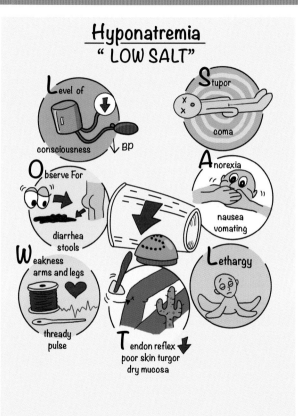

===== **What You Need to Know** =====

Hyponatremia—Low Salt

GENERAL

The Low Salt acronym is a mnemonic to help you remember the signs and symptoms of hyponatremia. Think of the words, 'Low Salt' as a visual image that will help you remember the important signs and symptoms.

When serum sodium levels are <135 mEq/L, hyponatremia is the resulting condition. It most often occurs when water intake increases, leading to a decreased sodium concentration.

The osmolarity of the ECF is lower than that of the ICF with hyponatremia, which causes water to move into the cell leading to cellular swelling, reduced cell function, and in severe cases, the cell will burst (lysis) and die.

ASSESSMENT: RECOGNIZE CUES

LOW SALT represents signs and symptoms of hyponatremia:
- **L**evel of consciousness - diminished
- **O**bserve for diarrhea
- **W**eakness in arms and legs, thready pulse
- **S**tupor, seizures, coma, death
- **A**norexia, nausea, vomiting
- **L**ethargy
- **T**endon reflex diminished, poor skin turgor, dry mucosa

NURSING MANAGEMENT: TAKE ACTION

- Monitor for cerebral changes (level of consciousness, lethargy), neuromuscular changes (tendon reflexed diminished; weakness), intestinal changes (diarrhea, anorexia, nausea, vomiting), and cardiovascular changes (thready pulse).
- Priority of care is monitoring the client's response to the treatment and *preventing hypernatremia and fluid overload.*
- Anticipate reduction in dosages of diuretics that lose sodium.
- Nutrition therapy includes increasing oral sodium intake and restricting oral fluid intake.

Important nursing implications	Serious/life-threatening implications
Most frequent side effects	Patient teaching

33

NURSING MANAGEMENT OF HYPONATREMIA

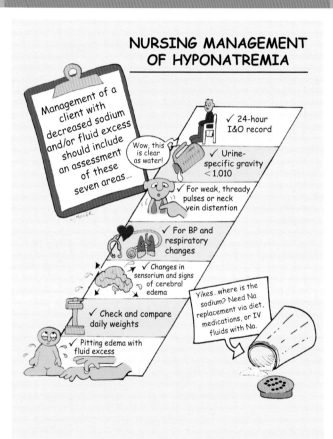

Fluids & Electrolytes

What You Need to Know
Management of Hyponatremia

MEDICAL MANAGEMENT: GENERATE SOLUTIONS

- Treat the underlying cause.
- Administer hypertonic solutions to restore sodium balance when hyponatremia is due to water excess (small volumes of 3% NaCl).
  - Too rapid correction of sodium can cause irreversible neurologic damage.
- Provide nutritional counseling.
- Increase foods containing sodium.
- Administer vasopressin receptor antagonists (conivaptan or tolvaptan) for the treatment of hyponatremia caused by fluid excess (dilutional).

NURSING MANAGEMENT: TAKE ACTION

- Closely monitor neurologic signs during sodium replacement.
- Obtain daily weights.
- Measure I&O—loss or gain of 4.4 lb is equal to 2 L of fluid.
- Check the color, consistency, and amount of urine. The urine should be a light straw color without sediment present.
- Monitor vital signs.
- Assess for intravascular overload during infusion of sodium solutions— tachypnea, tachycardia, and SOB.
- Teach the client how much fluid they are allowed per day and how to identify fluid retention.
- Increase oral sodium intake to restore sodium balance in mild hyponatremia.

Important nursing implications	Serious/life-threatening implications
Most frequent side effects	Patient teaching

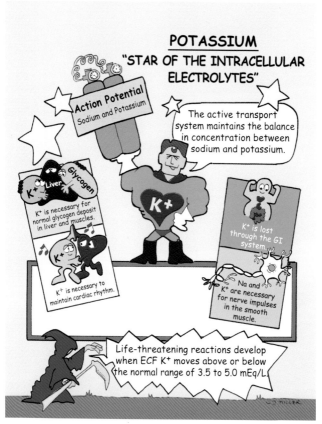

===== **What You Need to Know** =====

Potassium

SIGNIFICANCE OF POTASSIUM

Potassium is the most abundant cation found in ICF. Potassium regulates fluid balance and keeps osmolality within the ICF. Potassium also plays a key role in preserving normal cardiac rhythms and maintaining skeletal and smooth muscle contraction. Changes in serum pH levels also precipitate changes in serum potassium.

SOURCES OF POTASSIUM

- Bananas; dark green, leafy vegetables; raisins; and salt substitutes
- All-bran cereals, potatoes, and dried beef (beef jerky, dried fruit)

CONTROL OF POTASSIUM

Kidneys are the primary regulators of potassium. As the serum potassium level rises, so does the level in the renal tubules. A concentration gradient occurs, and potassium is lost in the urine.

Too much potassium in the ECF increases catecholamine levels, causing aldosterone levels to increase. Increased aldosterone levels cause the potassium to leave the ECF and travel into the kidneys (distal renal tubules) where it is excreted with urine.

Insulin can also lower the concentration of potassium by helping potassium travel into liver and muscle cells where it is used in the process of breaking down carbohydrates and proteins by moving glucose into the ICF.

Clients receiving increased amounts of insulin (total parenteral nutrition [TPN], diabetic ketoacidosis [DKA]) should have their potassium levels monitored closely because insulin may cause low levels of potassium.

FUNCTIONS OF POTASSIUM

- Maintains fluid balance in the cells
- Contracts skeletal, cardiac, and smooth muscles
- Helps breakdown carbohydrates and fats
- Promotes cellular growth
- Maintains acid-base balance

Important nursing implications	Serious/life-threatening implications
Most frequent side effects	Patient teaching

HYPERKALEMIA
SERUM POTASSIUM >5.1 mEq/L

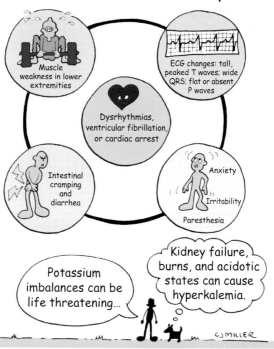

Muscle weakness in lower extremities

ECG changes: tall, peaked T waves; wide QRS; flat or absent P waves

Dysrhythmias, ventricular fibrillation, or cardiac arrest

Intestinal cramping and diarrhea

Anxiety

Irritability

Paresthesia

Kidney failure, burns, and acidotic states can cause hyperkalemia.

Potassium imbalances can be life threatening...

CJ MILLER

Fluids & Electrolytes

======== **What You Need to Know** ========
Hyperkalemia

GENERAL

The normal serum potassium levels are 3.5 to 5.0 mEq/L. When the potassium level is >5.1 mEq/L, the condition is known as *hyperkalemia.*

- Potassium levels between 5.1 and 6.0 mEq/L are considered to be *mild hyperkalemia.*
- Potassium levels of 6.1 to 7.0 mEq/L are considered to be *moderate hyperkalemia,* and levels above 7 mEq/L reflect *severe hyperkalemia.*

  Hyperkalemia most commonly occurs as a result of excessive potassium intake combined with the body's inability to excrete potassium.

  Acute kidney failure, Addison disease, and interstitial nephritis, secondary to diabetes mellitus will decrease the excretion of potassium.

  Ingestion of potassium-containing foods in clients with kidney failure and the administration of IV potassium may also cause increased serum potassium levels.

  Cardiovascular changes are the most severe problems of hyperkalemia and are the most common cause of death in clients with hyperkalemia.

ASSESSMENT: RECOGNIZE CUES

- Muscle cramps and twitching in early stage of hyperkalemia with tingling and burning sensations, followed by numbness in the hands and feet and around the mouth (paresthesia)
- As hyperkalemia progresses, muscle weakness occurs followed by flaccid paralysis.
  - Weakness moves up from the hands and feet and first affects the muscles of the arms and legs.
  - Respiratory muscles are not affected until serum potassium levels reach lethal levels.
- Diarrhea hyperactive bowel sounds, lethargy, fatigue
- Bradycardia, hypotension
- Cardiac dysrhythmias—ectopic beats heart block, ventricular fibrillation
- Electrocardiographic (ECG) changes

Important nursing implications	Serious/life-threatening implications
Most frequent side effects	Patient teaching

<u>MURDER</u>

SIGNS AND SYMPTOMS OF INCREASED SERUM K⁺

M—Muscle weakness
U—Urine, oliguria, anuria
R—Respiratory distress
D—Decreased cardiac contractility
E—ECG changes
R—Reflexes, hyperreflexia, or areflexia (flaccid)

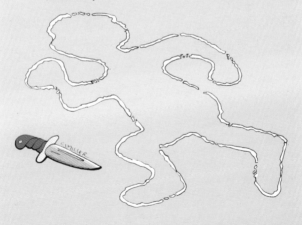

What You Need to Know
Hyperkalemia—MURDER

GENERAL

The normal serum potassium levels are 3.5 to 5.0 mEq/L. When the potassium level is >5.1 mEq/L, the condition is known as *hyperkalemia.* Hyperkalemia most commonly occurs as a result of excessive potassium intake combined with the body's inability to excrete potassium.

The acronym MURDER is used to trigger the symptoms that correspond to each letter of the word—**M**uscle weakness, **U**rine, **R**espiratory distress, **D**ecreased cardiac contractility, **E**CG changes, and **R**eflexes.

ASSESSMENT: RECOGNIZE CUES

- **M**uscle cramps in the extremities followed by weakness
- **U**rine, oliguria, and anuria (i.e., kidney disease leads to failure to eliminate potassium)
- **R**espiratory distress
- **D**ecreased cardiac contractility
- **E**CG changes
  - Tall, peaked T waves and flat or absent P waves
  - Shortened QT intervals
  - ST segment depression, prolonged PR interval, widened QRS complex
- **R**eflexes—hyperreflexia or areflexia (flaccid)

Important nursing implications	Serious/life-threatening implications
Most frequent side effects	Patient teaching

THE HYPERKALEMIA "MACHINE"
CAUSES OF INCREASED SERUM K+

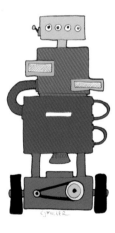

M	Medications—ARBs, ACE inhibitors, NSAIDs
A	Acidosis—Metabolic and respiratory
C	Cellular destruction—Burns, traumatic injury
H	Hypoaldosteronism, hemolysis
I	Intake—increased food, IV rate, salt substitute
N	Nephrons, kidney failure
E	Excretion—Impaired

What You Need to Know
Hyperkalemia—MACHINE

GENERAL

The MACHINE acronym (**M**edications, **A**cidosis, **C**ellular destruction, **H**ypoaldosteronism, **I**ntake, **N**ephrons, **E**xcretion) can be used to trigger memory association with the symptoms corresponding to each letter of the word.

The normal serum potassium levels are 3.5 to 5.0 mEq/L. When the potassium level is >5.1 mEq/L, the condition is known as *hyperkalemia*. Hyperkalemia most commonly occurs as a result of excessive potassium intake combined with the body's inability to excrete potassium.

CAUSES OF HYPERKALEMIA: GENERATE SOLUTIONS

- **M**edications—angiotensin-converting enzyme (ACE) inhibitors, angiotensin receptor blockers (ARBs), nonsteroidal antiinflammatory drugs (NSAIDs), and potassium-sparing diuretics
- **A**cidosis—metabolic and respiratory
- **C**ellular destruction—burns, traumatic injury, tumor lysis syndrome, and tissue catabolism (fever, sepsis)
- **H**ypoaldosteronism and hemolysis
- **I**ntake—excessive potassium from foods and salt substitutes, IV infusion of potassium, and potassium supplements
- **N**ephrons—kidney failure
- **E**xcretion—impaired

Important nursing implications	Serious/life-threatening implications
Most frequent side effects	Patient teaching

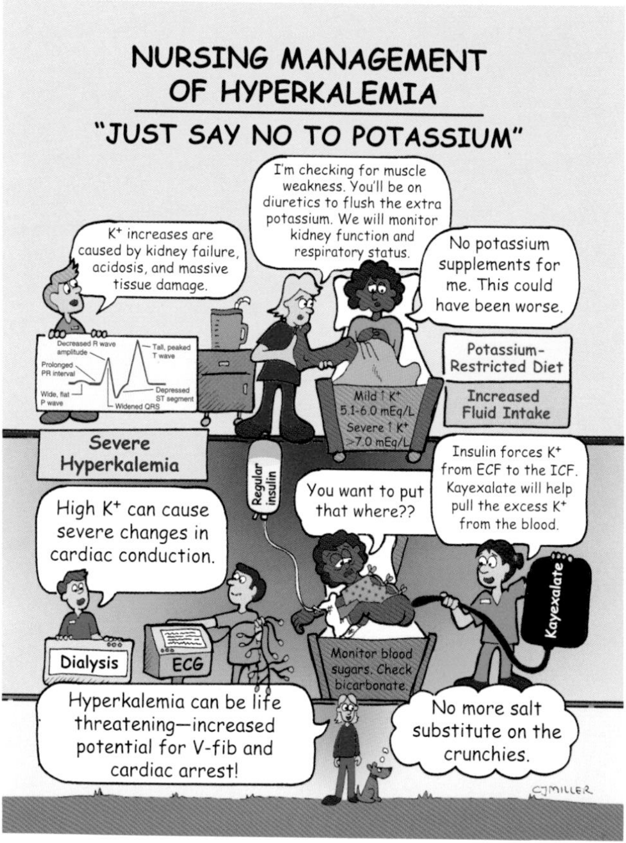
NURSING MANAGEMENT OF HYPERKALEMIA
"JUST SAY NO TO POTASSIUM"
K+ increases are caused by kidney failure, acidosis, and massive tissue damage.
I'm checking for muscle weakness. You'll be on diuretics to flush the extra potassium. We will monitor kidney function and respiratory status.
No potassium supplements for me. This could have been worse.
Decreased R wave amplitude
Tall, peaked T wave
Prolonged PR interval
Wide, flat P wave
Widened QRS
Depressed ST segment
Potassium-Restricted Diet
Increased Fluid Intake
Mild ↑ K+ 5.1-6.0 mEq/L
Severe ↑ K+ >7.0 mEq/L
Severe Hyperkalemia
Regular insulin
You want to put that where??
Insulin forces K+ from ECF to the ICF. Kayexalate will help pull the excess K+ from the blood.
High K+ can cause severe changes in cardiac conduction.
Kayexalate
Dialysis
ECG
Monitor blood sugars. Check bicarbonate.
Hyperkalemia can be life threatening—increased potential for V-fib and cardiac arrest!
No more salt substitute on the crunchies.
CJMILLER

Management of Hyperkalemia

MEDICAL MANAGEMENT: GENERATE SOLUTIONS

- Eliminate potassium intake, both orally and via IV.
- Promote excretion of potassium by administering diuretic agents.
- Initiate dialysis if the client is in kidney failure.
- Assess and administer Kayexalate, when needed, to treat mild-to-moderate hyperkalemia. Kayexalate is an ion-exchange resin that exchanges sodium ions for potassium ions in the intestine and excretes the potassium via the feces.
- Administer IV insulin to push potassium from the ECF to the ICF. It may be given with glucose to prevent rebound hypoglycemia.
- Assess and administer, if needed, IV sodium bicarbonate if hyperkalemia is secondary to acidosis.
- Immediately administer IV calcium gluconate to the client experiencing cardiac dysrhythmias, secondary to life-threatening potassium levels.

NURSING MANAGEMENT: TAKE ACTION

- Assess cardiac status at least q2h due to the risk of heart rate falling below 60 beats/min or the appearance of spiked T waves.
- Assess dietary potassium intake.
- Monitor kidney function (urine output and laboratory values).
- Teach the client that the use of ACE inhibitors and potassium-sparing diuretic agents will cause increased serum levels of potassium.
- Teach the client to limit the amount of foods containing potassium (leafy vegetables, salt substitutes, dried fruits, bananas, and cantaloupe).
- Teach the client the signs and symptoms of hyperkalemia and about the need to report them immediately to the healthcare provider.
- Provide continuous ECG monitoring to monitor for dysrhythmias while the client is in the hospital.
- Monitor blood sugar (BS) levels with insulin administration.

Important nursing implications	Serious/life-threatening implications
Most frequent side effects	Patient teaching

HYPOKALEMIA
"WHEN IS POTASSIUM TOO LOW?"
(SERUM K+ <3.5 mEq/L)

Respiratory alkalosis

Metabolic alkalosis via diuretic use and ↑ urine output

Watch labs and look for symptoms of low potassium.

Nasogastric suction

Severe vomiting and diarrhea

Symptoms include skeletal muscle weakness in the legs, the smooth muscles of the GI system, and weakness or paralysis of the respiratory muscles. The main cardiac issue of hypokalemia is potentially lethal ventricular dysrhythmias.

An estimate of total body potassium loss is calculated to establish the amount to be replaced.

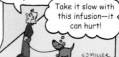

Take it slow with this infusion—it can hurt!

Fluids & Electrolytes

=== **What You Need to Know** ===
Hypokalemia

GENERAL

When the serum potassium level is <3.5 mEq/L, the condition is known as *hypokalemia*. The main cause of hypokalemia occurs from abnormal losses in the body, such as diuresis. During diuresis, potassium is excreted with urine because of high aldosterone levels. Thiazides and loop diuretic agents are the primary causes of hypokalemia. Corticosteroids and beta-adrenergic antagonists can increase potassium loss.

A direct relationship exists between low magnesium levels and low potassium levels. Low magnesium levels stimulate the release of renin, which causes an increase in aldosterone levels and the excretion of potassium.

GI losses (i.e., diarrhea, vomiting, gastric suctioning, ostomy fluids) can lower potassium levels.

Other conditions that may cause low potassium levels are DKA, metabolic alkalosis, and pernicious anemia.

ASSESSMENT: RECOGNIZE CUES

- Fatigue and weakness (early signs)
- Leg cramps (early sign)
- Weak, irregular pulse
- Hyperglycemia caused by the impaired release of insulin
- Decreased GI motility—nausea, vomiting, and paralytic ileus
- Bradycardia
- ECG changes
  - Flattened T wave, eventual emergence of a prominent U wave
  - ST segment depression, a slightly peaked P wave
  - Frequent premature ventricular contractions (PVCs)
  - Inability to concentrate urine and diuresis (with prolonged hypokalemia)

DIAGNOSTIC FINDINGS

- Serum potassium <3.5 mEq/L

Important nursing implications	Serious/life-threatening implications
Most frequent side effects	Patient teaching

Hypokalemia

" 7-Ls"

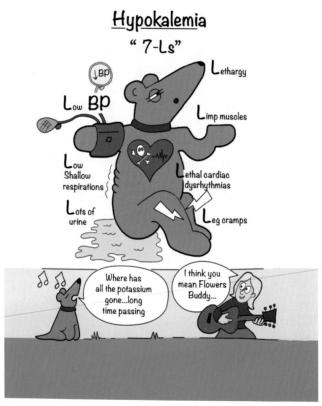

What You Need to Know
Hypokalemia—7 L's

GENERAL

The acronym 7 L's is a mnemonic to help you remember the signs and symptoms of hypokalemia. Think of the words that start with an 'L' as a visual image that will help you remember the important signs and symptoms.

When serum potassium levels are <3.5 mEq/L, hypokalemia is the resulting condition, which can be a life-threatening condition. It most often occurs with the loss of potassium from the GI tract (diarrhea, vomiting, nasogastric suctioning, ileostomy drainage), kidney (diuretics, hyperaldosteronism, magnesium deficiency), and skin (diaphoresis). Other mechanisms of potassium loss include a shift of potassium into the cells due to increased insulin release (associated with an IV dextrose load), insulin therapy (diabetic ketoacidosis), alkalosis, increased levels of epinephrine (stress), and lack of potassium intake (starvation, diet low in potassium, and lack of potassium added to parenteral fluids when client is NPO).

ASSESSMENT: RECOGNIZE CUES

The 7 L's represent signs and symptoms of hypokalemia:
- **L**ow blood pressure
- **L**ow shallow respirations
- **L**ots of urine
- **L**ethargy
- **L**imp muscles
- **L**ethal cardiac dysrhythmias
- **L**eg cramps

Important nursing implications

Most frequent side effects

Serious/life-threatening implications

Patient teaching

NURSING MANAGEMENT OF HYPOKALEMIA

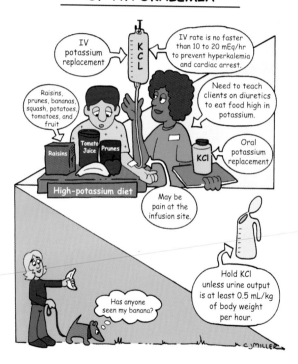

What You Need to Know
Management of Hypokalemia

MEDICAL MANAGEMENT: GENERATE SOLUTIONS

- Administer potassium chloride (KCl) supplements when clients are taking loop or thiazide diuretic agents and digitalis to help prevent hypokalemia.
- Assess and administer potassium orally or via IV.
  - When given via IV, potassium may cause irritation and pain at the site. Central lines are the preferred site for IV administration.
  - Preferred levels for serum potassium are 3.5 to 5 mEq/L.
  - KCl should not exceed the IV rate of 10 to 20 mEq/L per hour. Recommended infusion rate is 5 to 10 mEq/L per hour. Rapid infusion could cause hyperkalemia and cardiac arrest.
- Hypokalemia will increase the action of digitalis.

NURSING MANAGEMENT: TAKE ACTION

- Assess respiratory status at least q2h due to the risk of respiratory insufficiency.
- If given orally, encourage the client to take the KCl supplement with a full glass of water to promote absorption in the GI tract.
- Never give potassium IV push; it may be fatal.
- Never administer KCl unless there is adequate urine output—at least 0.5 mL/kg of body weight.
- Monitor the IV site for phlebitis or infiltration; KCl is irritating to the veins.
- Monitor the client on digoxin for signs of digoxin toxicity.
- Teach the client to recognize the signs and symptoms of hypokalemia and the need to report them immediately to the physician.
- For clients taking diuretic agents, explain the importance of increasing potassium intake in the diet.
- Teach the client about foods that are high in potassium.
- Teach the client that salt substitutes contain 50 to 60 mEq/L of potassium and should be avoided if the client is taking a potassium-sparing diuretic agent.
- Explain the need for a follow-up visit to have serum potassium levels drawn for those at risk.

Important nursing implications	Serious/life-threatening implications
Most frequent side effects	Patient teaching

CALCIUM
"HOW MUCH IS ENOUGH?"

Total body calcium is about 1200 g.

Calcium is the major cation for the structure of the bone and teeth.

99% of calcium is in the bone and teeth. The rest is in plasma and ECF.

Serum calcium in the blood is 9 to 10.5 mg/dL.

Calcium works as an enzyme co-factor for clotting and hormone secretion.

It also maintains plasma membrane stability and permeability, especially of the cardiac cell nerve receptors.

Calcium aids in the transmission of nerve impulses and contraction of muscles.

CJMILLER

=== **What You Need to Know** ===
Calcium

SIGNIFICANCE OF CALCIUM

Calcium is commonly found in bones and teeth and is the most abundant mineral found in the body. Calcium helps maintain muscle tone, hormone secretion, transmission of nerve impulses, and contraction of skeletal and heart muscles.

SOURCES OF CALCIUM

Calcium is commonly found in the following products:
- Dairy products—milk, cheese, yogurt, sour cream, cottage cheese, and ice cream
- Canned salmon, sardines, and oysters
- Fruit juices labeled "fortified"
- Dark green, leafy vegetables—spinach, kale, rhubarb, collard greens, and broccoli

CONTROL OF CALCIUM

Calcium is controlled by parathyroid hormone (PTH), vitamin D, and calcitonin. PTH is excreted by the parathyroid gland when low levels of serum calcium are present. PTH helps move calcium out of the bones, increasing GI reabsorption of calcium in the ileum and renal tubule reabsorption of calcium. Vitamin D is necessary to absorb calcium from the GI tract. Calcitonin is produced by the thyroid gland and excreted when high levels of serum calcium are found. Calcitonin does the exact opposite of PTH because it tries to prevent absorption of calcium and promote excretion through the renal tubules. If an increase in calcium exists, then most often a decrease in phosphate is observed, and vice versa.

FUNCTIONS OF CALCIUM

- Is necessary for the development of strong teeth and bones
- Helps maintain muscle tone
- Contributes to the regulation of BP by maintaining cardiac contractility
- Is an enzyme co-factor in the clotting cascade; assists in forming blood clots with the release of thromboplastin from platelets
- Is necessary for nerve transmission and contraction of skeletal and cardiac muscles

Important nursing implications	Serious/life-threatening implications
Most frequent side effects	Patient teaching

HYPERCALCEMIA
"TOO MUCH CALCIUM!"

Back with the facts! Serum calcium levels >10.5 mg/dL are too much. Causes are hyperparathyroidism, cancers with bone metastases, Paget's disease, hyperthyroidism, or thiazide diuretics.

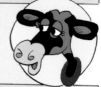

Hypercalcemia causes a loss of excitability in cell membranes and fatigue, weakness, lethargy, anorexia, nausea, constipation, and kidney stones from increased calcium salts.

ECG activity may show shortened QT interval and depressed T waves, bradycardia, and varying degrees of heart block.

I want to be a cow when I grow up.

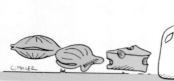

What You Need to Know
Hypercalcemia

GENERAL

- Several factors can cause hypercalcemia; however, in the majority of cases, hyperparathyroidism is the cause.
- Increased intake of vitamin D (overdose) can cause elevated calcium levels.
- Malignancies from the destruction of bones by tumor invasion in breast and lung cancer and multiple myeloma account for hypercalcemic symptoms.
- Prolonged immobilization leads to elevated serum calcium levels from bone loss.
- Rarely does hypercalcemia occur because of increased calcium intake, such as ingestion of antacids containing calcium or after excessive IV administration during a cardiac arrest.
- Thiazide diuretic agents can increase calcium levels.

ASSESSMENT: RECOGNIZE CUES

- Anorexia, nausea, and vomiting
- Fatigue, lethargy, and confusion
- Constipation, abdominal distention, and abdominal pain
- Hypoactive bowel sounds or absent bowel sounds
- Polyuria
- Dehydration
- Weakness and depressed reflexes
- ECG changes
  - Shortened QT interval and ST segment
  - Depressed T wave
  - Bradycardia
  - Heart block

DIAGNOSTIC FINDINGS

- Serum calcium level >10.5 mg/dL

| Important nursing implications | Serious/life-threatening implications |
| Most frequent side effects | Patient teaching |

NURSING MANAGEMENT OF HYPERCALCEMIA

- Loop diuretics
- Calcium chelators
- ↑ Hydration to 3000 to 4000 mL to flush calcium and to ↓ calculi formulation

The treatment for hypercalcemia is to promote the excretion of calcium in urine.

Synthetic calcitonin can be given to lower calcium levels.

Monitor I&O, vital signs, muscle weakness, and heart rate and rhythm.

What You Need to Know
Management of Hypercalcemia

MEDICAL MANAGEMENT: GENERATE SOLUTIONS

- Administer IV fluids, followed by a loop diuretic agent, that is, furosemide. (The excretion of calcium is followed by the excretion of sodium.)
- Administer bisphosphonates (pamidronate, etidronate) to help reduce bone resorption.
- Administer calcitonin via IV to promote kidney excretion of calcium.
- Administer calcium chelators (calcium binders), such as plicamycin and penicillamine.
- Treat nausea with antiemetic medications.
- Give stool softeners for constipation.

NURSING MANAGEMENT: TAKE ACTION

- Encourage the client to increase their oral intake of fluids to 3 to 4 L/day.
- Institute safety precautions for the client at risk for injury.
  - Be aware of an altered gait and weakness.
  - Assess neurologic status every 2 to 4 hours—loss of consciousness (LOC) and orientation.
- Encourage increased mobility.
- Monitor for dysrhythmias—tachycardia (mild hypercalcemia) and bradycardia (severe hypercalcemia).
- Monitor IV site for infiltration, erythema, and pain.
- Teach the client to limit their intake of foods high in calcium.
  - Avoid vitamin preparations that contain vitamin D.
- Hypercalcemia increases clotting times; there is an increased risk for thrombosis formation with venous stasis.

Important nursing implications	Serious/life-threatening implications
Most frequent side effects	Patient teaching

HYPOCALCEMIA

Hypocalcemia occurs when serum Ca++ concentrations are less than 9.0 mg/dL...and this is how it can happen.

Inadequate dietary intake

Inadequate absorption

Deposition of ionized calcium in bone or soft tissue

Too much dietary phosphorus that binds with calcium

Parathyroid

Decrease in PTH and lack of vitamin D

• Confusion
• Irritability
• Palpitations
• Numbness and tingling in hands, toes, and lips.
• Restlessness

Mild   Severe
Symptoms

• Convulsions
• Intestinal muscle involvement (diarrhea)
• Tetany
• Prolonged bleeding time
• Hypotension
• Prolonged Q-T interval
• Dysrhythmias

What You Need to Know
Hypocalcemia

GENERAL

Hypocalcemia can occur as a result of malignancies, vitamin D deficiency, acute pancreatitis, decreased intake of calcium-containing foods, increased intake of phosphorus (antacids), administration of a large amount of stored blood products, and removal of the parathyroid gland (loss of PTH). Hypocalcemia may also develop because of an excessive loss of calcium with the use of diuretic agents.

ASSESSMENT: RECOGNIZE CUES

- Painful muscle spasms or cramps occur in the calf muscles or foot during sleep or rest ("charley horses").
- **Tetany.** Is initially characterized by numbness and tingling of the nose, ears, and fingertips (paresthesias). (It may progress to painful muscle spasms and convulsions.)
- **Positive Chvostek sign.** Twitching of the cheek occurs in response to tapping the facial nerve. (Think C for *Chvostek* = cheek.)
- **Positive Trousseau sign.** Carpal spasm of the hand develops when a BP cuff is inflated above the systolic pressure for several minutes.
- Hyperreflexia is observed.
- Abdominal cramping and diarrhea.
- Skeletal changes with chronic states include osteoporosis.
- Laryngospasm develops.
- Dysrhythmias (ventricular tachycardia or fibrillation, torsades de pointes [prolonged QT interval], and elongation of ST segment) can occur.
- Severe hypotension.
- Hypomagnesemia frequently occurs.

DIAGNOSTIC FINDINGS

- Serum calcium level <9.0 mg/dL

Important nursing implications	Serious/life-threatening implications
Most frequent side effects	Patient teaching

59

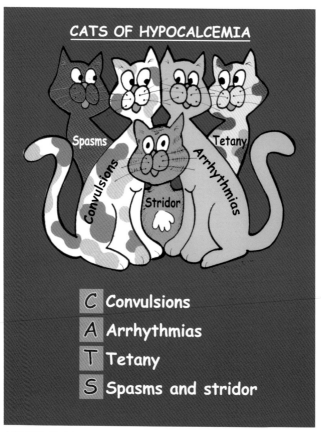

What You Need to Know
Hypocalcemia—CATS

GENERAL

Hypocalcemia can occur because of malignancies, vitamin D deficiency, decreased intake of calcium-containing foods, increased intake of phosphorus (antacids), administration of blood products, acute pancreatitis, and removal of the parathyroid gland.

Using the acronym CATS (**C**onvulsions, **A**rrhythmias, **T**etany, **S**pasms) helps establish a memory-triggering device to bring the serious signs and symptoms to mind.

ASSESSMENT: RECOGNIZE CUES

- **C**onvulsions (seizures), confusion, and paresthesias
- **A**rrhythmias (ventricular fibrillation, torsades de pointes [prolonged QT interval], and elongation of ST segment)
- **T**etany and hyperreflexia
- **S**pasms and laryngospasm with stridor
- **Positive Chvostek sign.** Twitching of the cheek in response to tapping the facial nerve (Think *C* for *Chvostek* = cheek.)
- **Positive Trousseau sign.** Carpal spasm of the hand when a BP cuff is inflated above the systolic pressure for several minutes
- Severe hypotension

Important nursing implications	Serious/life-threatening implications
Most frequent side effects	Patient teaching

NURSING MANAGEMENT OF HYPOCALCEMIA

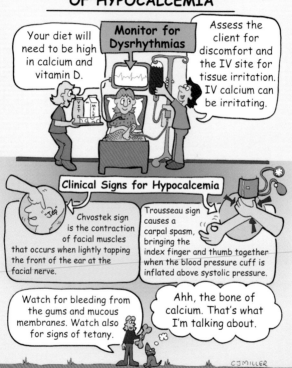

Fluids &
Electrolytes

What You Need to Know
Management of Hypocalcemia

MEDICAL MANAGEMENT: GENERATE SOLUTIONS

To manage nonacute hypocalcemia medically:
- Administer calcium carbonate by mouth with vitamin D to help absorb calcium in the GI tract.
- Administer magnesium if the client's serum levels are low.

To manage acute hypocalcemia in an emergency setting:
- Administer calcium gluconate or calcium chloride (CaCl) by slow IV push.

NURSING MANAGEMENT: TAKE ACTION
- Monitor serum calcium levels every 4 to 6 hours. The goal is to maintain calcium levels between 7 and 9 mg/dL (titrate drip accordingly).
- Assess IV site for infiltration:
  - Calcium gluconate and CaCl are damaging to tissue, which can lead to tissue necrosis.
- Monitor cardiac rhythm and ECG changes.
- Assess for decreasing BP.
- Evaluate for the presence of paresthesia.
- Check for Chvostek and Trousseau signs.
- Avoid rapid IV push administration, which could lead to a rapid drop in BP, dysrhythmias, and cardiac arrest.
- Do not administer intramuscularly (IM) because doing so causes local pain and may lead to tissue sloughing and necrosis.
- Initiate seizure precautions.
- Initiate injury prevention strategies with chronic hypocalcemia (bones are brittle and fragile, and may fracture easily).

Important nursing implications	Serious/life-threatening implications
Most frequent side effects	Patient teaching

PHOSPHORUS

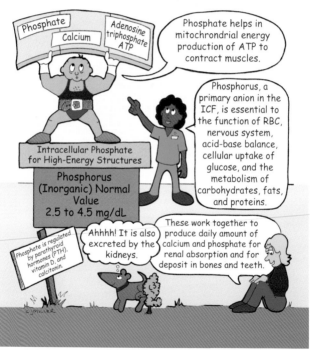

--- **What You Need to Know** ---
Phosphorus

SIGNIFICANCE OF PHOSPHORUS

Phosphorus is an essential mineral found in every cell of the human body. It is the second most abundant mineral next to calcium, accounting for roughly 1% of the body's total weight. It is deposited with calcium for bone and tooth structure, with 85% found primarily in the bone.

SOURCES OF PHOSPHORUS

- Milk, cheese, and eggs
- Meat, fish, fowl, nuts, legumes, and dried fruit

CONTROL OF PHOSPHORUS

A reciprocal relationship exists between phosphorus and calcium (when phosphate is elevated, then calcium is low). Just as calcium needs vitamin D for absorption in the GI tract, so does phosphorus. Phosphate is involved as the primary constituent in the mitochondrial energy production of adenosine triphosphate (ATP). (Note: *phosphate* is part of the word.) ATP is used as an energy storage medium for the body.

Maintenance of normal phosphorus balance requires adequate kidney functioning because the kidneys are the primary route for phosphate excretion. A small amount of phosphate is lost in the feces.

PTH is also important in maintaining normal levels of phosphorus by altering the kidney's reabsorption of phosphorus and the shift of phosphorus from the bones to the plasma.

FUNCTIONS OF PHOSPHORUS

- Keep bones and teeth healthy
- Intermediary in the metabolism of protein, carbohydrates, and fats
- Acid-base buffering
- Acidification of the urine
- Role in the formation of DNA and RNA
- Muscle contraction (it provides the energy in the form of ATP)
- Production of phospholipids (helps form structure of the cell membrane)
- Proper function of red blood cells

HYPERPHOSPHATEMIA

=== **What You Need to Know** ===
Hyperphosphatemia

GENERAL

The major condition that leads to an elevated level of phosphorus (hyperphosphatemia) in the body is acute or chronic renal failure. Other causes include hypoparathyroidism, increased intake of foods high in phosphorus (milk), excessive use of laxatives or enemas containing phosphate (Fleet enema), large intakes of vitamin D (which increase GI absorption of phosphorus), and chemotherapy for certain malignancies (lymphomas). Phosphorus is added to processed foods. The blood absorbs almost all the added phosphorus in processed foods and only absorbs about 20% - 50% of the phosphorus in natural foods like meat and eggs. Phosphorus from animal sources has a higher absorption rate than that from plants.

ASSESSMENT: RECOGNIZE CUES

- Reciprocal relationship to calcium exists. A high phosphorus level relates to a low calcium level, which leads to hypocalcemia.
  - Tetany and twitching of muscles, especially of the hands and feet
  - Tingling, numbness, and cramps
  - Nervousness, irritability, and apprehension
  - Anorexia, nausea, and vomiting
  - Tachycardia, dysrhythmias, and conduction problems
- Deposition of calcium-phosphorus precipitates in skin, soft tissue, cornea, viscera, and blood vessels.

DIAGNOSTIC FINDINGS

- Serum phosphate >4.5 mg/dL (1.5mmol/L)

Important nursing implications	Serious/life-threatening implications
Most frequent side effects	Patient teaching

NURSING MANAGEMENT OF HYPERPHOSPHATEMIA

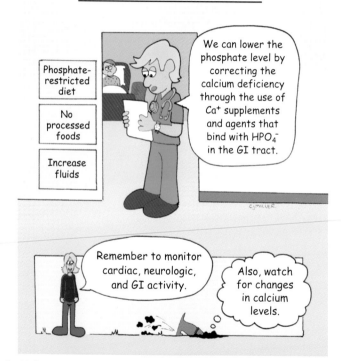

Phosphate-restricted diet

No processed foods

Increase fluids

We can lower the phosphate level by correcting the calcium deficiency through the use of Ca^+ supplements and agents that bind with HPO_4^- in the GI tract.

Remember to monitor cardiac, neurologic, and GI activity.

Also, watch for changes in calcium levels.

===== **What You Need to Know** =====
Management of Hyperphosphatemia

MEDICAL MANAGEMENT: GENERATE SOLUTIONS

- Administer vitamin D preparations such as calcitriol (Rocaltrol) in oral preparations, calcitriol injection (Calcijex) for IV administration, or paricalcitriol (Zemplar) to treat hyperphosphatemia caused by kidney failure, secondary to hyperparathyroidism.
- If hyperphosphatemia is related to volume depletion or respiratory or metabolic acidosis, treat the underlying condition first to correct the phosphate excess.
- Administer calcium-free phosphate binders, such as sevelamer hydrochloride (Renagel), sevelamer carbonate (Renvela), and lanthanum carbonate (Fosrenol), which reduce absorption of dietary phosphate from the GI tract. (*Note: Sevelamer hydrochloride can cause metabolic acidosis, whereas sevelamer carbonate may not.*)
- Administer calcium-based phosphate binders, such as calcium carbonate (Os-Cal, Caltrate) and calcium acetate (PhosLo), which are used to bind phosphate in the bowel.
- Aluminum-based antacids promote the elimination of phosphate from the GI tract by binding with phosphate (aluminum hydroxide) but are used with caution with clients with kidney failure.
- Cinacalcet (Sensipar), a drug to control PTH excess, is also used to manage hyperphosphatemia.

NURSING MANAGEMENT: TAKE ACTION

- Assess for constipation, which can be caused by taking phosphate binders.
- Assess for signs of hypocalcemia (tetany) because of the reciprocal relationship between phosphate and calcium.
- Monitor serum phosphate and calcium levels.
- Teach the client to limit foods high in phosphate—milk, cheese, egg yolk, meat, fish, fowl, nuts, and processed foods. Most foods that are high in phosphate are also high in calcium.
- Teach the client that fruits and vegetables are low in phosphate, especially spinach, rhubarb, bran, and whole grain foods, which may be increased.
- Teach the client to avoid phosphate-containing substances, such as laxatives and enemas.

HYPOPHOSPHATEMIA
LESS THAN 2.5 mg/dL IS PHOSPHATE DEFICIENCY

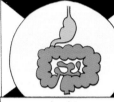

Intestinal malabsorption

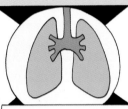

Severe respiratory alkalosis

A lack of phosphate interferes with oxygen transported by red blood cells and energy metabolism

ECG: Extreme muscle wasting may cause respiratory failure, cardiomyopathies, and bradycardia

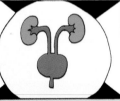

Increased excretion of phosphate

Altered nerve and muscle function causes irritability, confusion, numbness, coma, and convulsions.

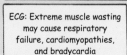

What You Need to Know
Hypophosphatemia

GENERAL

Hypophosphatemia is most commonly caused by intestinal malabsorption related to Vitamin D deficiency and increased kidney excretion of phosphate (as a result of hyperparathyroidism) and rarely is due to low dietary intake. It may also occur in respiratory alkalosis and during parenteral nutrition with inadequate phosphate replacement. The intake of phosphate-binding antacids (aluminum- and magnesium-based antacids), long-term alcohol abuse, diarrhea, and malabsorption syndromes can lead to hypophosphatemia. A reciprocal relationship occurs between phosphate and calcium (i.e., when phosphate levels are low, then calcium levels are high).

ASSESSMENT: RECOGNIZE CUES

Acute symptoms result from a sudden decrease in phosphate; chronic symptoms occur when the loss is gradual.

- Neurologic symptoms: Acute—irritability, confusion, numbness, seizures, and coma. Chronic—memory loss and lethargy
- Decreased strength: Acute—difficulty speaking, weakness of respiratory muscles, which can lead to possible respiratory failure. Chronic—lethargy, weakness, joint stiffness, rickets, and osteomalacia
- Decreased myocardial contractility with decreased cardiac output (dysrhythmias, heart failure) and hypotension
- Rhabdomyolysis—due to depletion of ATP and inability of muscles to maintain membrane integrity
- Clients at risk for hypophosphatemia include preterm newborns (can lead to calcium deficiency and osteopenia of prematurity), X-linked hypophosphatemic rickets, and those with severe malnutrition

DIAGNOSTIC FINDINGS

- Serum phosphate <2.5 mg/dL

SOURCES OF PHOSPHATE

- Meats, especially organ meats
- Fish and poultry
- Milk and milk products, ice cream, cheese, and yogurt
- Whole grains, legumes, and nuts

NURSING MANAGEMENT OF HYPOPHOSPHATEMIA
"TWO LEVELS OF CARE"

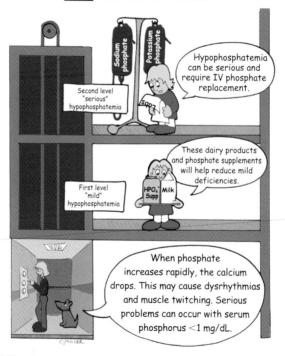

What You Need to Know
Management of Hypophosphatemia

MEDICAL MANAGEMENT: GENERATE SOLUTIONS

- Treatment for mild deficiency
  - Increase intake of foods high in phosphorus (meat, fish, poultry, dairy products).
  - Take oral phosphorus supplements.
- Treatment for severe deficiency
  - Administer an IV infusion of sodium phosphate or potassium phosphate when serum phosphate is < 1 mg/dL.

NURSING MANAGEMENT: TAKE ACTION

- Assess and document changes in LOC and orientation.
- Teach the client that neurologic changes are temporary.
- Closely monitor the rate of infusion of IV phosphorus.
- During IV replacement, monitor serum calcium and phosphate levels every 6 to 12 hours.
- Monitor for sudden hypocalcemia and hyperkalemia, secondary to calcium phosphate binding, as a complication of IV phosphate administration.
- Provide cardiac monitoring during the infusion of phosphate because of the increased risk of dysrhythmias, hypotension.
- Assess for hypoxemia because clients on ventilators are at higher risk for developing hypophosphatemia.
- Evaluate mobility and the presence of bone pain.

| Important nursing implications | Serious/life-threatening implications |
| Most frequent side effects | Patient teaching |

MAGNESIUM
A MAJOR INTRACELLULAR CATION

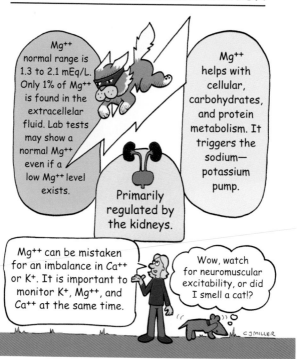

Mg^{++} normal range is 1.3 to 2.1 mEq/L. Only 1% of Mg^{++} is found in the extracellelar fluid. Lab tests may show a normal Mg^{++} even if a low Mg^{++} level exists.

Mg^{++} helps with cellular, carbohydrates, and protein metabolism. It triggers the sodium—potassium pump.

Primarily regulated by the kidneys.

Mg^{++} can be mistaken for an imbalance in Ca^{++} or K^+. It is important to monitor K^+, Mg^{++}, and Ca^{++} at the same time.

Wow, watch for neuromuscular excitability, or did I smell a cat!?

CJMILLER

What You Need to Know

Magnesium: A Major Intracellular Cation

SIGNIFICANCE OF MAGNESIUM

Magnesium plays an important role in intracellular reactions, bone metabolism, and nerve-action potentials. It activates enzymes for carbohydrate and protein metabolism. It also triggers the sodium-potassium pump and affects the levels of potassium in the cell. Magnesium is important in the normal function of the central nervous system (CNS) and in the cardiac system.

SOURCES OF MAGNESIUM

- Vegetables (best source, especially green)
  - Broccoli, spinach, squash, avocados, and potatoes
- Whole grains, nuts, and seeds (especially pumpkin and chia seeds)
- Because magnesium is a mineral, commonly found in tap water
- Fruits (bananas and oranges)
- Peanut butter and dark chocolate

CONTROL OF MAGNESIUM

Although it is not quite understood which organs control the levels of magnesium in the body, the kidneys help control high magnesium levels by excreting it through the feces and conserving it by storing it in bone when levels are low. A direct relationship exists among magnesium, potassium, and calcium. This relationship is important because only 1% of magnesium is found in the ECF. Serum laboratory values may reveal a normal magnesium level even if a low ICF magnesium level exists.

FUNCTIONS OF MAGNESIUM

- Is a co-enzyme in the metabolism of carbohydrates and proteins
- Acts directly on the myoneural junction, affecting muscular irritability and contractions
- Maintains strong and healthy bones

Important nursing implications	Serious/life-threatening implications
Most frequent side effects	Patient teaching

HYPERMAGNESEMIA

"TOO MUCH OF A GOOD THING IS A BAD THING."

Normal range for adults is 1.3 to 2.1 mEq/L

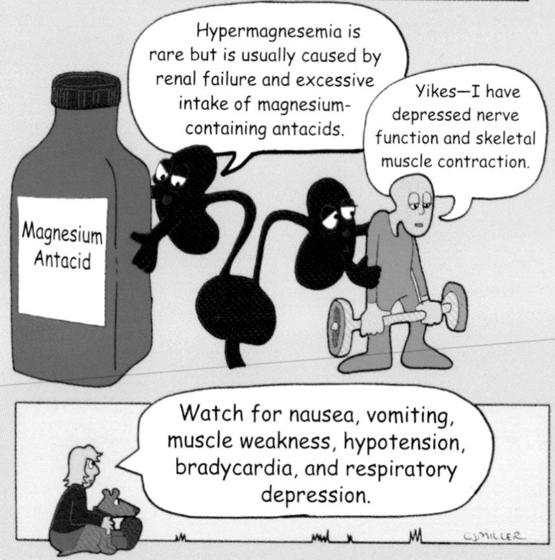

Hypermagnesemia

GENERAL

Occurs with magnesium levels >2.1 mEq/L. This condition is most often seen in clients with kidney failure. Decreased muscle activity is seen as a result of a blockage of acetylcholine at the myoneural junction; respiratory muscles may be affected, as well as cardiac conduction.

Hypermagnesemia may also be seen in clients with diabetes mellitus, DKA, hypothyroidism, or adrenal insufficiency.

Clients who ingest large amounts of magnesium-containing antacids such as Tums, Maalox, or Mylanta, or laxatives such as Epsom salt, Milk of Magnesia (MOM), and citrate of magnesia, are also at increased risk for developing hypermagnesemia. Women with preterm labor and severe preeclampsia receiving IV magnesium sulfate can develop hypermagnesemia.

ASSESSMENT: RECOGNIZE CUES

- Muscular weakness, confusion, and drowsiness (mild elevation)
- Nausea, vomiting, constipation, and headache
- Decreased deep tendon reflexes and blurred vision
- Greatly elevated level of serum magnesium is a medical emergency.
  - Client will exhibit absent deep tendon reflexes, decreased LOC, bradycardia, and severe hypotension, which may result in coma and cardiac arrest.

DIAGNOSTIC FINDINGS

- Check BUN and creatinine routinely.
- Serum magnesium level is >2.1 mEq/L.
- When obtaining a blood sample, it should not be shaken because this may cause hemolysis of red blood cells, which may give a false positive of an elevated magnesium level.

Important nursing implications	Serious/life-threatening implications
Most frequent side effects	Patient teaching

NURSING MANAGEMENT OF HYPERMAGNESEMIA

TX with compromised kidneys...

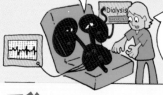

We were already failing—why did we take all those magnesium antacids?

Dialysis

It's important to teach clients about the hazards of using over-the-counter products that contain magnesium.

TX with healthy kidneys...

If the kidneys are okay, then pour in fluids to ↑ excretion of magnesium and ↓ serum levels.

In emergency situations, an IV calcium preparation may be given to oppose the effects of magnesium on cardiac muscles.

Closely monitor serum laboratory levels, ECG, and cardiac and neurologic assessments.

Watch the K⁺—it goes up too!

What You Need to Know
Management of Hypermagnesemia

MEDICAL MANAGEMENT: GENERATE SOLUTIONS

- Administer IV solution containing calcium salts (calcium gluconate) for severe hypermagnesemia.
- Administer loop diuretics (e.g., furosemide) for clients with normal kidney function.
- Discontinue use of medications containing magnesium.
- Clients with kidney failure or impaired kidney function may be dialyzed.

NURSING MANAGEMENT: TAKE ACTION

- Assess neurologic status for mental status and reflexes.
- Report if the client has absent deep tendon reflexes (especially the patellar reflex) or decreasing LOC.
- Closely monitor I&O and kidney function.
- If kidney function is adequate, increased fluids and diuretics promote urinary excretion of magnesium
- Anticipate dialysis if kidney function is inadequate.
- Monitor vital signs; watch for bradycardia and hypotension.
- Provide a list of foods and drugs containing magnesium that should be avoided.
- Provide continuous cardiac monitoring for the client with elevated levels.
  - Report a prolonged QT interval, a wide QRS complex, or the presence of an atrioventricular (AV) block.
- Keep in mind that the half-time elimination of magnesium is approximately 28 hours.
- Carefully monitor serum magnesium levels in obstetric clients receiving magnesium sulfate for the treatment of preeclampsia and preterm labor.
- Evaluate the newborn's magnesium levels if the mother received magnesium sulfate immediately before delivery.
- Teach client to avoid excessive use of magnesium containing antacids and laxatives.

Important nursing implications	Serious/life-threatening implications
Most frequent side effects	Patient teaching

HYPOMAGNESEMIA
"THE HYPOMAGNESEMIA SEVEN"

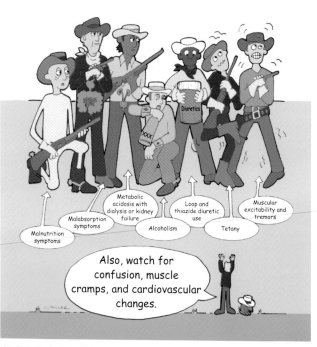

Fluids &
Electrolytes

What You Need to Know
Hypomagnesemia

GENERAL

Normal serum laboratory values for magnesium are 1.3 to 2.1 mEq/L. When magnesium levels fall below 1.3 mEq/L, the condition is known as *hypomagnesemia*. Knowing the clients who are at risk for developing this condition is imperative. Magnesium deficiency also can cause hypocalcemia, as the two are interrelated.

Hypomagnesemia may be present in clients with malabsorption disorders such as inflammatory bowel disease (IBD), celiac disease, bowel resection, and following gastric bypass surgery. Other causes of hypomagnesemia may be observed in the client going through alcohol withdrawal, acute pancreatitis, and severe malnutrition.

Clients receiving diuretics (loop and thiazide), proton pump inhibitors, insulin, amphotericin B, aminoglycosides (e.g., gentamicin, tobramycin, neomycin), or chemotherapeutic agents (cisplatin, cyclosporine), are at increased risk for developing hypomagnesemia.

ASSESSMENT: RECOGNIZE CUES

- Signs and symptoms are similar to those of hypocalcemia.
- Increased neuromuscular ability (secondary to hypocalcemia)
  - Leg and foot cramping
  - Tremors and hyperactive deep tendon reflexes
  - Twitching (positive Chvostek and Trousseau signs)
  - Tetany and seizures
- Cardiac dysrhythmias (atrial fibrillation and frequent PVCs, torsades de pointes, and ventricular fibrillation)
- Difficulty swallowing, constipation, and abdominal distention
- Paralytic ileus (with severe hypomagnesemia)

DIAGNOSTIC FINDINGS

- Magnesium serum laboratory value is <1.3 mEq/L.
- Calcium levels may be decreased because of decreased action of PTH.
- Potassium levels may be decreased because of a failure of the sodium-potassium pump.
- Symptoms may not be seen in the client until magnesium levels are <1 mEq/L.

NURSING MANAGEMENT OF HYPOMAGNESEMIA

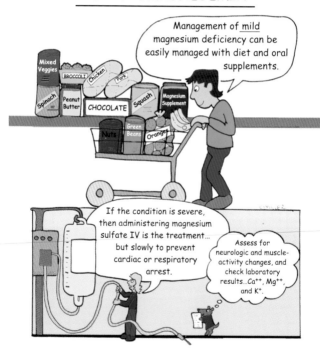

Management of _mild_ magnesium deficiency can be easily managed with diet and oral supplements.

If the condition is severe, then administering magnesium sulfate IV is the treatment… but slowly to prevent cardiac or respiratory arrest.

Assess for neurologic and muscle-activity changes, and check laboratory results…Ca^{++}, Mg^{++}, and K^+.

What You Need to Know
Management of Hypomagnesemia

MEDICAL MANAGEMENT: GENERATE SOLUTIONS

- Replace magnesium either orally or parenterally.
- For oral replacement, assess and administer magnesium oxide tablets or antacids containing magnesium (e.g., Mylanta, Maalox, Tums).
- Assess and correct potassium and calcium levels.
- For IV replacement therapy, administer magnesium sulfate via an infusion pump.
  - Infuse magnesium sulfate at a slow rate (<150 mg/min).
  - For symptomatic, severe hypomagnesemia in a stable client with adequate kidney function, 1 to 2 grams of magnesium sulfate may be given over 1 hour.
  - Never give magnesium as an IV bolus; it may cause sudden cardiac arrest.

NURSING MANAGEMENT: TAKE ACTION

- Obtain a history of the current medications the client is taking. Certain medications may need to be discontinued if they are contributing to low magnesium levels.
- If the client is given IV magnesium, check for decreased patellar reflexes (DTRs), respiratory difficulty, and decreasing BP prior to administration and while infusing. Stop the infusion if these occur.
- Assess for the presence of dysphagia.
- Assess serum laboratory values for the presence of hypokalemia and hypocalcemia.
- Provide a list of magnesium-rich foods to the client, such as green vegetables, beans, peas, nuts, seeds, unrefined grains.
- Advise the client that diuretics may be discontinued.
- Keep in mind that the client with low magnesium levels clinically resembles the client with low calcium levels.

Important nursing implications	Serious/life-threatening implications
Most frequent side effects	Patient teaching

ACID-BASE BALANCE

Too many H+ make more acid. The body works with a very narrow range. Small pH changes alter biologic processes.

Most diseases can cause an imbalance. An imbalance can cause more problems than the disease itself.

I am the first to respond to keep the pH in balance and to neutralize the H+.

#1 Buffy Buffer

HYDROGEN
H+

pH = hydrogen ion (H+) concentration in solution

↓ pH = acidic = ↑ H+

↑ pH = alkalotic = ↓ H+

If Buffy can't handle it, then I step in to control CO_2.
↑ CO_2 = ↑ H_2CO_3 (carbonic acid).

#2 Respiratory System

I'm slow but dependable. I control bicarbonate (HCO_3^-) to neutralize it.

#3 Kidney System

Normal pH by Body Fluid	
Gastric juices	1 to 3
Urine	5 to 6
Arterial blood	7.35 to 7.45
Venous blood	7.31 to 7.41
CSF	7.32
Pancreatic fluid	7.8 to 8

--- **What You Need to Know** ---

Acid-Base Balance

GENERAL

The concentration of hydrogen (H⁺) ions controls the acid-base balance in the body. The higher the concentration of H⁺, the lower the pH and the more acidic is the solution. The lower the concentration of the H⁺, the higher the pH and the more alkaline is the solution. The normal range for the body pH is from 7.35 to 7.45. The normal acid-base ratio is 1:20 — 1 part carbon dioxide (CO_2) to 20 parts bicarbonate (HCO_3^-). If this balance is altered, then either a state of acidosis or alkalosis exists.

CONTROLLERS OF THE pH

1st response: The body buffers are HCO_3^-, phosphate, protein, and ammonium. These buffers are present in body fluids and respond immediately to buffer or combine with excess base or acid produced during normal metabolism. This buffering maintains a normal pH level. However, the effect of these buffers is limited and depends on adequate functioning of the respiratory and kidney systems.

 2nd response: The respiratory center of the brain responds to changes in levels of H⁺ by controlling the CO_2 via the respiratory response. CO_2 + water (H_2O) = carbonic acid. If too many H⁺ ions exist, then the respiratory rate increases to eliminate excessive CO_2, which decreases the H⁺.

 3rd response: The kidney or metabolic system regulates the H⁺ by increasing or decreasing the concentration of HCO_3^- and by increased excretion of H⁺.

- Acid-base balance is evaluated by an arterial blood gas (ABG) analysis.
- Normal ABG values are as follows:
  - pH — 7.35 to 7.45
  - Partial pressure of carbon dioxide in arterial blood ($PaCO_2$) — 35 to 45 mm Hg
  - Partial pressure of oxygen in arterial blood (PaO_2) — 80 to 100 mm Hg (reflects respiratory status but does not contribute to pH balance)
  - Oxygen saturation — 96% to 100%
  - Base excess: +1 to −2
  - Serum HCO_3^-: 22 to 26 mEq/L

Important nursing implications	Serious/life-threatening implications
Most frequent side effects	Patient teaching

ACIDOSIS

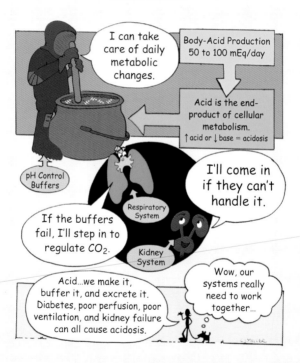

What You Need to Know

Acidosis

GENERAL

A state of acidosis exists when the pH is <7.35. It can be caused by problems in either the respiratory system (too much CO_2) or the metabolic system (too little HCO_3^-):

- **Respiratory acidosis (retention of CO_2):** Depression of the respiratory center (head injury, anesthesia, narcotic overdose), obstruction of respiratory passages (pneumonia, atelectasis), and chronic respiratory problems (chronic obstructive pulmonary disease [COPD]) prevent the normal excretion of CO_2 through ventilation.

- **Metabolic acidosis (deficit or loss of base HCO_3^- or excessive acid production):** Diabetic ketoacidosis (DKA), kidney failure, lactic acidosis (shock, cardiac arrest), and loss of HCO_3^- through diarrhea or intestinal fistulas. In these conditions, an excessive loss of HCO_3^- or alkaline fluids occurs.

  Serum potassium (K^+) tends to go up with acidosis. K^+ ions move from the intracellular fluid (ICF) to the extracellular fluid (ECF). The kidney tends to retain K^+ as it increases the secretion of H^+. When acidosis is corrected, K^+ will shift back into the cellular compartment (ICF). An increase in serum K^+ can result in dysrhythmias.

COMPENSATORY MECHANISM

Both the kidney and the lungs have a compensatory mechanism to assist the other organs when problems occur. The compensatory mechanism attempts to restore the 1:20 ratio of acid-to-HCO_3^- and return the pH to within normal limits (7.35 to 7.45).

  The compensatory mechanism is successful when the pH returns to normal; however, it does not mean the primary problem causing the imbalance has been resolved.

- If respiratory acidosis is the problem, then the kidneys will retain more HCO_3^- to compensate for the acidosis.
- If metabolic acidosis is the problem, then the lungs will increase excretion of CO_2 to assist the elimination of H^+ ions and compensate for the acidosis.

Important nursing implications	Serious/life-threatening implications
Most frequent side effects	Patient teaching

ALKALOSIS

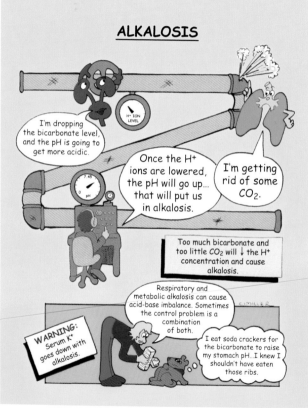

Acid-Base Balance

What You Need to Know
Alkalosis

GENERAL

A state of alkalosis exists when the pH is >7.45. It can be caused by problems in either the respiratory system (too little CO_2) or the metabolic system (too much HCO_3^-).

Respiratory alkalosis (loss of CO_2) tends to occur when people are nervous and breathe too rapidly (hyperventilation) and excrete excessive amounts of CO_2. It may also be caused by problems of the central nervous system (CNS) affecting the respiratory center.

Metabolic alkalosis is caused by an excessive retention of HCO_3^- or a loss of acid. It may occur if too much HCO_3^- has been given during resuscitation. It may also occur with gastric suctioning or prolonged vomiting and diarrhea.

K^+ tends to go down with alkalosis. K^+ moves into the cells (ICF) from the ECF, leading to hypokalemia. If alkalosis is corrected, K^+ will shift out of the ICF and back into the circulating volume (ECF).

COMPENSATORY MECHANISM

Both the kidney and the lungs have a compensatory mechanism to assist the other organs when problems occur. The compensatory mechanism attempts to restore the 1:20 ratio of acid to HCO_3^- and return the pH to within normal limits (7.35 to 7.45).

The compensatory mechanism is successful when the pH is within normal levels; however, it does not mean the primary problem causing the imbalance has been resolved.

- If respiratory alkalosis is the problem, then the kidneys will compensate by excreting more HCO_3^- to balance the pH.
- If metabolic alkalosis is a problem, the lungs will retain more CO_2 to balance the pH.

Important nursing implications	Serious/life-threatening implications
Most frequent side effects	Patient teaching

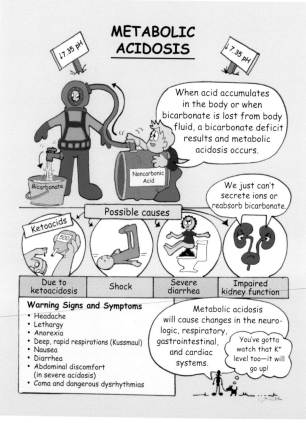

=== **What You Need to Know** ===
Metabolic Acidosis

SIGNIFICANCE OF METABOLIC ACIDOSIS

Metabolic acidosis occurs because of excess acid production in the body or rapid excretion of HCO_3^- from the body. When the metabolic system is the primary problem, the respiratory system compensates.

COMMON CAUSES OF METABOLIC ACIDOSIS

- Diabetic ketoacidosis (DKA) (most common)
- Lactic acidosis (shock, respiratory or cardiac arrest)
- Kidney failure
- Severe diarrhea
- Salicylate toxicity
- Starvation, dehydration
- Gastrointestinal (GI) fistulas, pancreatitis, and liver failure

ASSESSMENT: RECOGNIZE CUES

- Kussmaul respirations (deep, rapid respirations)
- Confusion, disorientation progressing to coma
- Headache and lethargy
- Hypotension, thready peripheral pulses
- Dysrhythmias secondary to hyperkalemia; bradycardia to heart block
- Warm flushed skin (peripheral vasodilation)
- Abdominal pain and nausea and vomiting

DIAGNOSTIC FINDINGS

ABG results will show the following:
- pH <7.35
- HCO_3^- <22 mEq/L
- Possible normal $PaCO_2$ (35 to 45 mm Hg). Respiratory compensation may occur, causing a decrease in the $PaCO_2$ level.
- Urine pH <6

| Important nursing implications | Serious/life-threatening implications |
| Most frequent side effects | Patient teaching |

NURSING MANAGEMENT OF METABOLIC ACIDOSIS

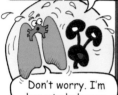

This acid is killing my kidneys.

Don't worry. I'm here to help you.

Nursing Management

Kidney function—check blood urea nitrogen (BUN), creatinine, and hemoglobin and hemocrit levels. Monitor hydration status for problems with fluid balance. Support respiratory function—turn, cough, and deep breathe. Check ABGs, and assess for Kussmaul respirations. Check electrolyte levels. K^+ usually goes up in acidosis; Ca^{++} usually goes down. Assess for cardiac dysrhythmias. Assess blood sugar levels; they may need to be corrected. Antidiarrheal medications and soda bicarbonate may be given to correct acidosis.

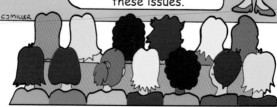

It is a nursing priority to assess and manage these issues.

Acid-Base Balance

What You Need to Know

Management of Metabolic Acidosis

MEDICAL MANAGEMENT: GENERATE SOLUTIONS

IV HCO_3^- may be administered in severe acidosis (if serum bicarbonate levels are low and the pH is <7.2); a rapid transition from acidosis to alkalosis can be detrimental.

- Frequently evaluate ABGs.
- Correct the precipitating cause of acidosis.

NURSING MANAGEMENT: TAKE ACTION

- Identify and treat the cause!
- Determine the history of the precipitating cause—diabetes, alcohol intake, renal disease, excessive GI fluid loss, and lactic acidosis.
- Assess serum laboratory results:
  - Blood urea nitrogen (BUN) and creatinine for kidney function
  - Serum electrolytes (K^+ tends to go up; may fluctuate with treatment.)
  - Serum glucose levels
- Monitor ABGs:
  - Check for a pH <7.35.
  - Check for a HCO_3^- <22 mEq/L.
- Monitor vital signs, including weight.
- If acidosis is a result of DKA, administer insulin. Watch for hypokalemia during the administration of insulin because insulin will assist K^+ to move into the cells (ICF).
- Give antiemetic medications for vomiting.
- Administer fluid replacement (0.9% or 0.45% sodium chloride [NaCl] for hydration therapy).
- Administer antidiarrheal medications if the cause is from excessive diarrhea.
  - Assess skin turgor, urine-specific gravity, and weight for hydration status.
  - Determine whether compensation is occurring. If the value (CO_2 or HCO_3^-) that does not match the direction of the pH is moving in the opposite direction, then compensation is occurring. Kidneys will compensate acidosis by increasing the HCO_3^-; lungs will compensate acidosis by decreasing the CO_2.

Important nursing implications	Serious/life-threatening implications
Most frequent side effects	Patient teaching

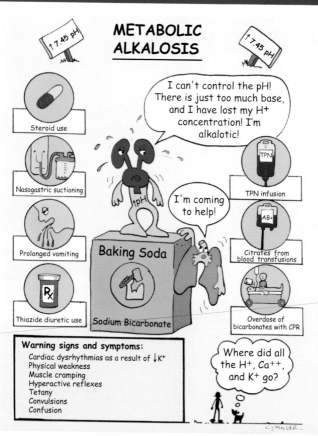

SIGNIFICANCE OF METABOLIC ALKALOSIS

Metabolic alkalosis occurs because of the loss of an acid or an increase in the level of HCO_3^- in the body. The lungs compensate by a decrease in respiratory rate to increase the level of plasma CO_2. The kidneys compensate by excreting more HCO_3^-

COMMON CAUSES

- Loss of acid through gastric suctioning or vomiting
- Excess alkali intake—antacids and sodium HCO_3^-
  - Adrenal disease (hyperaldosteronism)
  - Excessive intake of mineralocorticoids
- Diuretic therapy (high ceiling loop [furosemide] and thiazides)

ASSESSMENT: RECOGNIZE CUES

- Nervousness and dizziness
- Cardiac irritability—decreased K^+, ventricular dysrhythmias, and atrial tachycardia
- Nausea and vomiting
- Paresthesias in the fingers and toes
- Tetany and muscle cramps—late signs
- Hypoventilation (compensated by the lungs)
- Hydration status (tends to have a fluid volume deficit)

DIAGNOSTIC FINDINGS

- pH >7.45
- Normal PCO_2 (may increase because of compensation)
- HCO_3^- >26 mEq/L
- Urine pH >6

Important nursing implications	Serious/life-threatening implications
Most frequent side effects	Patient teaching

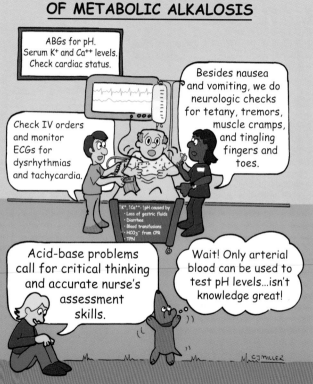

What You Need to Know
Management of Metabolic Alkalosis

MEDICAL MANAGEMENT: GENERATE SOLUTIONS

- Treat the precipitating cause.
- Stop the intake of HCO_3^-.
- For clients with GI fluid loss as a result of suctioning and vomiting, replace balanced fluids. Replace fluid lost from intestinal fistulas.

NURSING MANAGEMENT: TAKE ACTION

- Assess client to help identify the underlying problem.
- Evaluate client history for the precipitating cause—GI suctioning or vomiting.
- Monitor ABGs.
- Monitor K^+ values (hypokalemia usually occurs, but levels will increase with the treatment of alkalosis).
- If the client is taking digitalis, monitor pH, digitalis, and K^+ levels. Digitalis toxicity may occur with hypokalemia.
- Assess for dysrhythmias; tachycardia and dysrhythmias are related to decreased K^+.
- Monitor respirations; lungs will compensate by retaining CO_2.
- Give antiemetic medications to control nausea and vomiting.
- Assess for paresthesias (numbness and tingling) of toes and fingers.

Important nursing implications	Serious/life-threatening implications
Most frequent side effects	Patient teaching

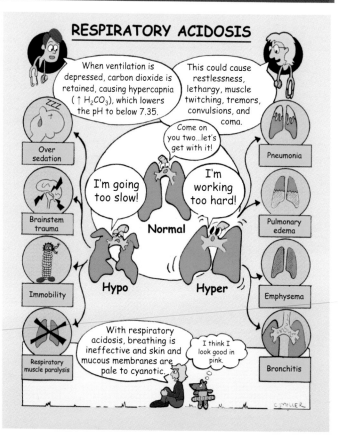

Respiratory Acidosis

SIGNIFICANCE OF RESPIRATORY ACIDOSIS

Respiratory acidosis occurs when an excess of CO_2 is in the blood. It is the most common of the acid-base imbalances.

COMMON CAUSES OF RESPIRATORY ACIDOSIS

Respiratory acidosis occurs secondary to problems that cause hypoventilation:
- CNS depression—head injury, sedatives, and anesthesia
- Increased resistance—aspiration, bronchospasm and laryngospasm, and prolonged narrowing of the airway (e.g., asthma, airway edema)
- Loss of lung surface—atelectasis, COPD, pneumonia, pneumothorax, and chronic pulmonary diseases
- Neuromuscular diseases affecting respiratory muscles—Guillain-Barré syndrome and myasthenia gravis
- Mechanical hypoventilation—increased retention of CO_2
- Opioid, sedative, or barbiturate overdose

ASSESSMENT: RECOGNIZE CUES

- Dyspnea
- Hypoventilation resulting in hypoxia
- Restlessness progressing to lethargy
- Drowsiness, confusion, and coma
- Tachycardia, tachypnea, and hypotension
- Dysrhythmias (ventricular fibrillation) associated with hypoxia and hyperkalemia
- Seizures
- Pale to cyanotic and dry skin
- Hypercapnia (elevated CO_2 level), which will cause cerebral vasodilation and increase problems with increased intracranial pressure (ICP).

DIAGNOSTIC FINDINGS

- pH is <7.35.
- PCO_2 is >45 mm Hg.
- HCO_3^- may be normal or increased because of compensation.
- Compensation from the renal system is slow.
- Urine pH is <6.

NURSING MANAGEMENT OF RESPIRATORY ACIDOSIS

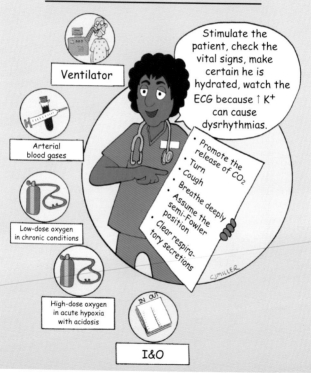

Management of Respiratory Acidosis

GENERAL

Although oxygen does not play a part in acid-base balance, acidosis will occur when the client does not have an adequate gas exchange. Respiratory suppression or hypoventilation, from whatever cause, will precipitate hypoxia (too little oxygen) and hypercapnia (too much CO_2). It is the excess CO_2 that causes the respiratory acidosis.

MEDICAL MANAGEMENT: GENERATE SOLUTIONS

- Administer bronchodilators.
- If the client is on a ventilator, it may be necessary to increase the tidal volume to facilitate maximum volume and gas exchange to increase expiration of CO_2.
- Correct the precipitating cause of hypoxia or respiratory problem if possible.

NURSING MANAGEMENT: TAKE ACTION

- Use semi-Fowler position to facilitate ventilation.
- Suction as needed to remove excessive mucus.
- Teach the client to use an incentive spirometer.
- Encourage the client to turn, cough, and breathe deeply.
- Have an artificial airway available.
- Assess patency of the airway—respiratory rate and breath sounds.
- Assess for tachycardia secondary to hypoxia.
- Maintain a calm, reassuring attitude. (Clients with dyspnea or hypoxia [or both] tend to be restless and anxious.)
- Monitor the client for bradypnea (respiratory rate <12 breaths per minute).
- Initiate seizure precautions.
- Assess medications. (Sedation may need to be decreased.)
- Encourage ambulation. (Assess client's response to activity. Stop activity with increasing shortness of breath [SOB] and tachycardia.)

Important nursing implications	Serious/life-threatening implications
Most frequent side effects	Patient teaching

RESPIRATORY ALKALOSIS

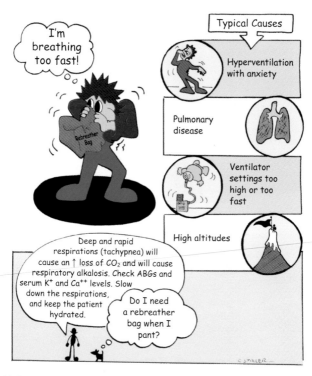

Acid-Base Balance

What You Need to Know
Respiratory Alkalosis

GENERAL

Respiratory alkalosis occurs when the client hyperventilates, causing an excessive loss of CO_2. *Hypocapnia* is the term used to describe decreased levels of CO_2. The condition is most commonly seen in clients who are hyperventilating secondary to hypoxia as a result of acute pulmonary conditions. Most often, the decrease in CO_2 occurs rapidly and does not allow time for kidney compensation to occur. Clients with chronic respiratory alkalosis may have some kidney compensation.

COMMON CAUSES

- Hyperventilation syndrome (anxiety, fear, and hysteria)
- Hyperventilation is caused by:
  - Hypoxia
  - Pulmonary emboli
  - Pain
  - Fever
  - CNS problems (encephalitis and head injury)
  - Mechanical hyperventilation (tidal volume is too high and respiratory rate is too rapid)

ASSESSMENT: RECOGNIZE CUES

- Hyperventilation (hyperpnea)—hallmark sign
- Possible lightheadedness
- Dysrhythmias and tachycardia (K^+ may be decreased)
- Confusion
- Epigastric pain and nausea
- Numbness in fingers and toes (may progress to tetany or seizures)

DIAGNOSTIC FINDINGS

- pH >7.45
- PCO_2 <35 mm Hg
- HCO_3^- often within normal range (slow compensation)
- pH urine >6

Important nursing implications	Serious/life-threatening implications
Most frequent side effects	Patient teaching

NURSING MANAGEMENT OF RESPIRATORY ALKALOSIS

Kidneys help compensate for ↑ pH that occurs in respiratory alkalosis by retaining more H^+ ions.

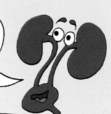

You can increase the retention of CO_2 by breathing into a paper bag or using a rebreather mask. Sedatives can also help in a crisis.

As with all acid-base imbalances, it is important to take these nursing actions...

Monitor:
- Respiratory rate and depth
- Tachycardia or ↓ BP
- Serum K^+ levels—cardiac dysrhythmias
- Hydration status—I&O

If the client is on digitalis, then check for toxicity.

Management of Respiratory Alkalosis

MEDICAL MANAGEMENT: GENERATE SOLUTIONS

- Assess the need for an antianxiety medication.
- If necessary, decrease the rate and tidal volume if the client is on a ventilator.

NURSING MANAGEMENT: TAKE ACTION

- Identify and correct precipitating cause.
- Monitor ABGs.
- Check for presence of decreased K^+; monitor for dysrhythmias.
- Try to relax or calm the client—encourage slow, deep breathing; may use relaxation techniques such as guided imagery.
- Encourage breathing into a paper sack or rebreathing mask to increase retention of CO_2.
- Reduce environmental noise and stimuli.
- Teach the client to slow down their respiratory rate.
- If the client is having pain, treat it with analgesic medications.
- If the client has a fever, administer antipyretic medications.

Important nursing implications	Serious/life-threatening implications
Most frequent side effects	Patient teaching

OVERVIEW OF SELECTED TRACE BODY MINERALS

Multimineral Mine

Minerals, electrolytes, and vitamins all play a major role in the quality of our overall physiology.

Iron and other minerals

Oxygen transport (iron)

Immune system protection (zinc)

Normal brain development and function (iron)

Neuro-transmitter function (iodine)

Synthesis of thyroid hormones T_3 and T_4 (iodine)

Minerals are absorbed in the small intestine. Problems there will cause an imbalance.

There's got to be gold in here somewhere!

Overview of Selected Trace Body Minerals

GENERAL

The *major minerals* are calcium, chloride, magnesium, phosphorus, potassium, sodium, and sulfur because they are needed in amounts greater than 100 mg/day. Iron, iodine, and zinc are *trace elements or minerals* found in small amounts in body tissue along with chromium, copper, fluoride, manganese, molybdenum, and selenium. Although the requirements for these trace minerals are small, they are a vital part in maintaining normal body functions. A well-balanced diet usually meets the daily requirements of minerals. However, deficiency and excess states can occur.

IRON

A majority of the body's iron is found in the hemoglobin of the red blood cells (RBCs) and represents approximately two-thirds of the iron found in the body. Hemoglobin is the oxygen-carrying protein in the RBCs. The remaining one-third of the iron is stored in the bone marrow, spleen, liver, and macrophages. Iron, B_{12}, and folic acid are necessary for the development of normal RBCs.

IODINE

Iodine is necessary for normal thyroid gland function. It is necessary for the body's metabolism and physical and mental development. Research is currently being conducted to identify the role of iodine in body tissue and other body functions. With a decrease of available iodine, the production of thyroid hormone (thyroxin) levels decreases. With a drop in the thyroid hormone, the production of the thyroid-stimulating hormone (TSH) increases. Iodine plays a role in the synthesis of the thyroid hormones T_3 and T_4 and in maintaining metabolism and nerve function, which is necessary for the action of osteoblasts in the production of collagen.

ZINC

Zinc plays a role in regulating the secretion of calcitonin from the thyroid gland, and it influences bone turnover. In addition, theories suggest that zinc is beneficial in preventing viral replication and in boosting the immune response. Zinc is also important in wound healing and sense of taste and smell.

Important nursing implications	Serious/life-threatening implications
Most frequent side effects	Patient teaching

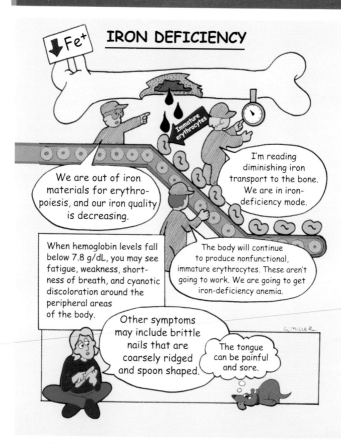

What You Need to Know
Iron Deficiency

GENERAL

A lack of dietary intake of iron, chronic blood loss, and excessive blood loss in hemorrhagic conditions can cause iron deficiency. As the liver and spleen destroy the old RBCs, the iron is recycled. If the stored iron is depleted, it will decrease the amount of hemoglobin produced. Chronic blood loss is the primary cause of iron deficiency in adults.

- **Pediatric implications of iron deficiency.** Normal-term infants have adequate iron storage for the first 5 to 6 months; premature infants may need an iron supplement at 2 to 3 months. Toddlers who drink more than 16 to 24 oz of cow's milk per day are at risk for developing iron deficiency. Cow's milk does not contain a significant amount of iron. When milk is taken with other foods, it may also decrease the ability of the body to absorb iron from food sources. Toddlers who drink a lot of milk tend to feel full and then do not want to eat other foods that contain iron. Adolescents are at risk because they are growing rapidly and have increased iron requirements. Girls who have started menses, especially if they have heavy menstrual blood loss, are also at increased risk of iron deficiency.
- **Older adult implications of iron deficiency.** Poor dietary intake, decreased absorption, and chronic blood loss should be considered.
- **Pregnancy implications.** Diversion of iron to the fetus for erythropoiesis, blood loss at delivery, and lactation can cause iron deficiency.

ASSESSMENT: RECOGNIZE CUES

- Pallor (skin, conjunctivae, sublingual)
- Glossitis (inflammation of the tongue)
- Fatigue, weakness, and headache
- Intolerance to cold temperatures
- Severe anemia—shortness of breath, dyspnea on exertion, tachycardia, and palpitations, which can progress to cardiac decompensation
- Chronic anemia in children (leads to growth retardation, developmental delay)
- "Spoon nails" (nails that develop in a concave shape) or vertical ridges

DIAGNOSTIC FINDINGS

- Hemoglobin levels <13 (men) to 12 (women) g/dL or two standard deviations below normal for age
- Low serum ferritin

IRON EXCESS—HEMOCHROMATOSIS

Wow...too much iron! Hemochromatosis (iron excess) is a genetic disorder. Increased absorption of Fe^+ deposited in soft tissue, especially in the liver, heart, and pancreas, can cause hepatomegaly and cirrhosis.

Watch for hyperpigmentation of the skin (bronzing), fatigue, cardiac dysrhythmias, cardiomyopathy, diabetes, and arthritis.

Treatment is done by drawing 500 mL of blood each week to drop the iron levels until stores are depleted. This may take 2 to 3 years.

I have a friend who has too much iron...they call him Rusty.

What You Need to Know

Iron Excess—Hemochromatosis

GENERAL

Iron excess is not as common as iron deficiency and is seen more frequently in men than in women. Iron excess has two forms: (1) genetic and (2) acquired. In acquired hemochromatosis, the most common cause is due to chronic blood transfusions used to treat thalassemia or caused by liver disease. The genetic disorder is an autosomal recessive disorder.

ASSESSMENT: RECOGNIZE CUES

- Early
  - Fatigue
  - Arthralgia
  - Impotence
  - Abdominal pain and weight loss
- Liver engorgement with hepatomegaly and cirrhosis
- Symptoms of diabetes
- Cardiomyopathy
- Changes in skin pigmentation
- Arthritis
- Testicular atrophy in men

DIAGNOSTIC FINDINGS

- Elevated serum ferritin
- Liver biopsy (definitive test for diagnosing)

MEDICAL MANAGEMENT: GENERATE SOLUTIONS

- Decrease serum iron levels by weekly removal of 500 mL of blood for 2 to 3 years until iron stores are depleted.
- Administration of chelation therapy with deferoxamine or deferasirox.

NURSING MANAGEMENT: TAKE ACTION

- Encourage client to limit intake of foods that are high in iron.
- Monitor vital signs during the removal of blood (phlebotomy).
- Provide care associated with monitoring for diabetes and cardiac failure.
- Iron excess frequently goes undiagnosed and untreated.

Important nursing implications	Serious/life-threatening implications
Most frequent side effects	Patient teaching

IODINE DEFICIENCY

What You Need to Know
Iodine Deficiency

GENERAL

Without sufficient iodine, the body is unable to synthesize the T_3 and T_4 thyroid hormones. The pituitary gland recognizes the decreased iodine state and releases the TSH. TSH stimulates the thyroid gland to synthesize and release more T_3 and T_4; both of which are necessary for the regulation of cellular metabolism and normal growth and development. Approximately 60% of the iodine in the body is stored in the thyroid gland. The remainder is found in the blood, ovaries, and muscle. Constant stimulation of the thyroid gland by the TSH will result in an increase in the size of the thyroid gland and may produce a goiter. The most devastating complications occur when iodine is deficient during fetal and neonatal growth.

ASSESSMENT: RECOGNIZE CUES

- Symptoms are frequently those associated with hypothyroidism—intolerance to cold, dry skin, weakness, lethargy, bradycardia, constipation, and enlargement of the thyroid gland (goiter).

DIAGNOSTIC FINDINGS

- Decreased T_4 and elevated TSH

MEDICAL MANAGEMENT: GENERATE SOLUTIONS

- Encourage the client to use iodized salt (70 mcg/g) in cooking and at the table to replace iodine.
- Initiate thyroid replacement therapy for symptoms of hypothyroidism.
- Remove the thyroid gland (thyroidectomy).

NURSING MANAGEMENT: TAKE ACTION

- Inform the client that 1 tsp of iodized salt is more than sufficient to satisfy the physiologic requirements for iodine intake.
- For clients on diets with severely restricted sodium intake, provide a list of foods (e.g., shellfish, yogurt, saltwater fish) that are recommended sources of iodine.
- Monitor thyroid function studies if the client is in the hospital.

Important nursing implications	Serious/life-threatening implications
Most frequent side effects	Patient teaching

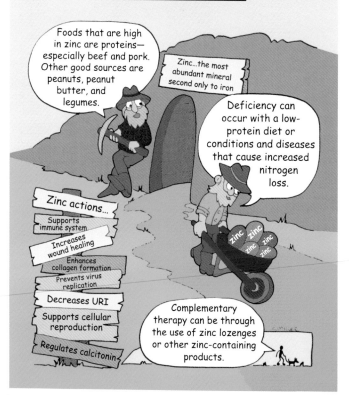

===== **What You Need to Know** =====
Zinc Deficiency

SIGNIFICANCE OF ZINC

Zinc deficiency may cause suppression of the immune system and result in increased opportunity for infection. Zinc is a necessary component for the normal functioning of the immune system and helps prevent replication of viruses and is involved in cell division, cell growth, and the breakdown of carbohydrates. Zinc also plays an important role in the catalytic activity of body enzymes, protein synthesis, and wound healing. Zinc is also needed for the senses of smell and taste. Risk factors for zinc deficiency include inadequate caloric intake, alcoholism, and diseases of the digestive tract. Oysters contain the highest level of zinc than any other food. Red meat, poultry, and beans also provide dietary zinc.

MEDICAL MANGAGEMENT: GENERATE SOLUTIONS

Zinc, vitamins A and C, and iron facilitate optimal wound healing. The dose of these elements may be higher than the recommended daily allowance.

Zinc may be used to prevent upper respiratory infections and skin disorders, as well as facilitate wound healing.

Supplements are available in oral tablets or lozenges. (Doses over 15 mg/day are not recommended.)

ASSESSMENT: RECOGNIZE CUES

Zinc deficiency may be characterized by growth retardation, anorexia, increased frequency of infections secondary to an impaired immune system, and delayed healing of wounds.

DIAGNOSTIC FINDINGS

Measuring the level of zinc in the body is difficult because zinc is present throughout the body as a component of proteins and nucleic acids.

NURSING MANAGEMENT: TAKE ACTION

- When taken for at least 5 months, zinc may reduce the risk of getting the common cold.
- Starting to take zinc supplements within 24 hours after cold symptoms begin may reduce how long the symptoms last and make the symptoms less severe.

Important nursing implications	Serious/life-threatening implications
Most frequent side effects	Patient teaching

TYPES OF IV THERAPY/SOLUTIONS, USES, AND PACKAGING

1000 mL

250 mL

500 mL

100 mL

250 mL

50 mL

Ladies and gentlemen, look around me. We have fluids and delivery bags and bottles for every purpose in every size. Choose them as ordered.

Hypertonic	Isotonic	Hypotonic
Osmolarity greater than body fluid	Osmolarity equal to body fluid	Osmolarity less than body fluid
Shifts fluid into the blood plasma by moving fluid from interstitial and ICF spaces.	Keeps fluid in the intravascular or plasma blood volume.	Shifts fluid from the plasma to the interstitial and ICF fluid.

These solutions are sterile. The containers should be checked for the expiration date, defects, leaks, and clarity.

Don't bite the bags!

The IV bags or bottles have calibration marks on the sides for fluid measurement. A bag has a soft plastic cap that must be removed before spiking to connect the tubing.

Expiration date

What You Need to Know

Types of Intravenous Fluids and Uses

ISOTONIC SOLUTIONS

Because isotonic solutions have the same osmolarity as normal body fluids (between 270 and 300 mOsm/L), isotonic solutions help by expanding the fluid in the extracellular fluid (ECF) space.

Examples: 0.9% normal saline (NS); lactated Ringer's (LR) solution; 5% dextrose in water (D_5W) and Ringer's solution

Common uses: Replacement of fluid loss and maintenance of fluid to keep the veins open with long-term intravenous (IV) administration

What to watch for:

Fluid volume overload

Low hemoglobin and hematocrit levels because of dilution by overexpansion of intravascular compartment

HYPOTONIC SOLUTIONS

Hypotonic solutions help hydrate the cells, can decrease the amount of fluid in the circulatory system (plasma fluid volume), and have an osmolarity less than 270 mOsm/L. Interstitial and intracellular (ICF) fluid volumes expand, and the plasma volume shrinks.

Example: 0.45% NS

Common uses: To lower serum sodium levels; to expand and hydrate cells

What to watch for:

Monitor sodium level.

Clients with low blood pressure are not usually given hypotonic solutions because doing so will further drop their blood pressure.

Hypotonic solutions have the potential to cause cellular swelling; monitor for changes in mental status that may indicate cerebral edema.

HYPERTONIC SOLUTIONS

Hypertonic solutions help restore circulating volume. An increased risk for both hypernatremia and volume overload of plasma or intravascular fluid exists.

Examples: 3% or 5% NaCl; D_5W ½ NS (D_5W 0.45% NS); D_5W 0.09% NS (D_5W NS) (*Note: the change in these hypertonic solutions is due to the rapid metabolization of the 5% dextrose.*)

Common uses: Hypovolemia and hyponatremia

What to watch for:
Wet breath sounds, increase in blood pressure
Fluctuation of serum sodium levels

Important nursing implications

Most frequent side effects

Serious/life-threatening implications

Patient teaching

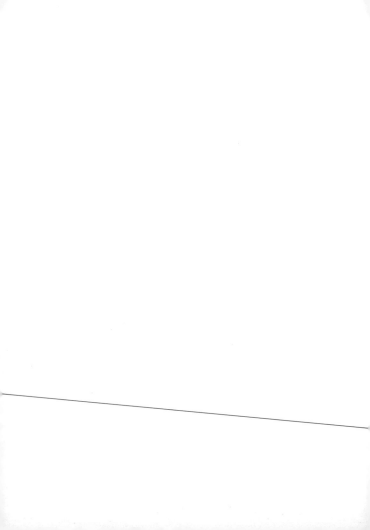

SELECTING ADMINISTRATION SETS

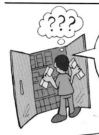

Hey, what kind of drop chamber, micro or macro? Vented or nonvented? Ports or without back-check valves? Buretrol or volutrol? How about roller valves and flow regulator attachments???

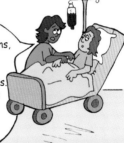

Micro (60 drops/min) are for kids and small infusions, so bring me a macro (10 to 15 drops/min). You only need a vented set for rigid plastic IV bags. The backports are for piggyback systems, and the volutrol is for small amounts. I'm not using a pump, so just the regular tubing is fine.

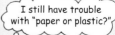

There are a lot of choices and things to consider when working with IV equipment.

I still have trouble with "paper or plastic?"

IV Therapy

What You Need to Know

Selecting Administration Sets

TYPES OF CONTAINER

- **Glass or Rigid Plastic.** Some specialty fluids come in glass containers that are vacuum sealed. Rigid IV containers require vented tubing to allow air to enter and displace the fluid as it leaves the container. (*Note: The use of glass IV containers is rare if not completely disappeared.*)
- **Plastic.** Most standard fluids come in flexible plastic containers. These require either regular or PediDrip tubing, but they do not require a vent.

ADMINISTRATION SETS

Drop Size
- Microdrop drip (PediDrip) chambers deliver 60 drops/min.
  - **Uses:** Pediatrics, older clients, and clients requiring limitations on IV infusion rate
- Macrodrop drip chambers deliver 10 to 15 drops/min.
  - **Uses:** Primarily adults; can be used to infuse fluids rapidly or to infuse a maintenance fluid (e.g., 125 mL/hr).

IV Ports
Continuous flow sets or lines are designed with a port to infuse secondary (piggyback) fluids, medications, or both.

Tubing
All tubing will require "priming" before connecting it to the client. No free air should be in the IV tubing.

IV Filters
IV filters are required for administering blood. Institution policies related to specific medications requiring filters should be checked.

Flow Control Devices
Roller clamps are designed to regulate the flow of fluid by applying pressure on the tubing.

Accessory Devices
These regulatory accessory devices surround the tubing and control the drip rate more effectively than the standard roller clamp.

IV infusion pumps
IV infusion pumps have the highest degree of accuracy for the delivery of specific volume of fluids on medications that must infuse at a specific rate.

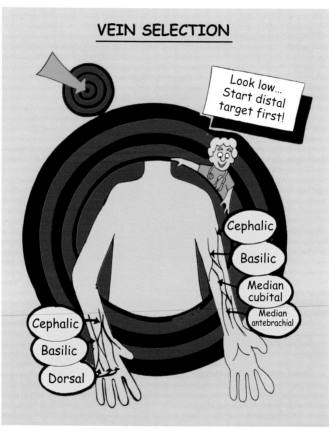

What You Need to Know
Vein Selection

NURSING IMPLICATIONS: TAKE ACTION

- Verify the order for the rate of IV fluid delivery.
- Check for allergies to latex (nurse's glove used in insertion) and iodine solutions or other solutions used to cleanse the skin.
- Verify the client with two forms of identification.
- Teach the client to limit use and mobility of the arm with the IV.

VEIN SELECTION

- Begin by inspecting the distal veins of the hands and arms.
- Preferably, use a vein on the client's nondominant side.
- Examine the cephalic vein in the hand and forearm and the median veins of the forearm.
- Select a vein that is straight and not previously used for IV insertion.
- Palpate the vein; it should be soft, full, and unobstructed.
- Avoid areas where valves exist in the veins (seen as small nodules in the vein). Threading a catheter through a vein valve is sometimes difficult.
- Avoid the veins of the hand in older clients (poor skin turgor) and in active patients receiving infusion therapy in the home or clinic.
- Select a vein that is appropriate for the type of solution and catheter required—select larger veins for blood or IVs that will stay in place for several days and for infusion of irritating fluids; for example, potassium and antibiotics are very irritating to tissue.
- For "butterfly" needles and short-term therapy, select suitable veins in the hands.
- Avoid the following:
  - Areas of flexion
  - Areas of previous infiltration or phlebitis
  - Veins on a surgically compromised limb (e.g., client who has recently had a mastectomy or has lymphedema)
  - Veins on side of the body that have been neurologically compromised (e.g., stroke; paralysis)
  - Veins in an extremity where circulation is compromised
  - Veins on the palmar side of the wrist because the median nerve is close to the area
  - Arm with a dialysis graft or fistula

VENIPUNCTURE DEVICE SYSTEMS

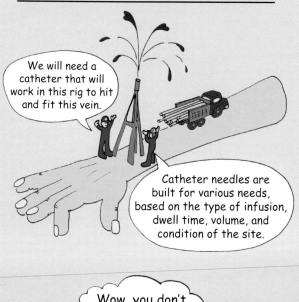

What You Need to Know

Venipuncture Device Systems

WINGED CATHETERS (BUTTERFLY NEEDLE)

Winged catheters consist of a stainless steel needle with soft pliable "wings" on either side to stabilize the needle in the vein and are associated with a high frequency of infiltration.

Uses: Short-term infusion of fluids or IV push medication

OVER-THE-NEEDLE CATHETERS

The over-the-needle catheter is a hollow tube that is threaded over the top of a needle or stylet. The needle is used to puncture the vein; blood appears in the flashback chamber when the vein is entered, and the catheter is then threaded over the needle into the vein. The flexible catheter is left in the vein and is the most common type used. The Centers for Disease Control and Prevention (CDC) recommend changing every 72 to 96 hours or if complications occur.

Uses: Infusion of IV fluids over several hours to days

MIDLINE CATHETERS

The midline catheter is 3 to 8 inches long and may be single or double lumen and is considered a type of "inside-the-needle" catheter. They are inserted into the upper arm with the aid of ultrasound guidance. The tip of the catheter resides no farther than in a peripheral vein (cephalic or basilic).

Uses: For IV therapy over 6 days and up to 14 days. Should not be used for vesicant medications, and blood should not be drawn from them.

CATHETER GAUGES

The smaller the number, the larger the catheter and needle diameter.
- 24 to 26 gauge—may be used on infants and older adults
- 22 gauge—most commonly used for general IV infusion
- 14 to 18 gauge—used in emergency situations or when large amounts of fluid must be infused rapidly, and blood transfusions

NURSING CONSIDERATIONS FOR THE SELECTION OF AN IV DEVICE: TAKE ACTION

- Amount of fluid and how long it will be infusing
- Viscosity of fluid (blood will infuse through a 22-gauge needle, but it will infuse more rapidly through an 18- or 20-gauge needle)
- Size and condition of the vein (the smallest catheter that will provide the flow rate ordered for the fluid is used)

IV INFUSION PUMPS

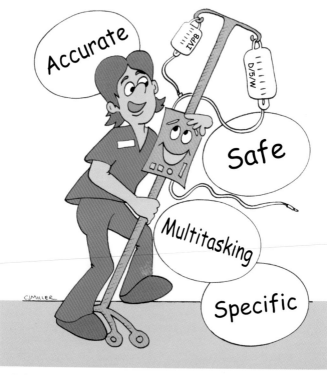

What You Need to Know

IV Equipment and Infusion Regulation Devices (IV Pumps)

MECHANICAL GRAVITY DEVICES

The nurse manually sets the infusion rate on a dial or control device (i.e., roller clamp or other type of control device) that is located on the line. These devices may be used in outpatient settings or for short-term infusions and should *not* be used for infants and children because accuracy of delivery cannot be guaranteed.

ELECTRONIC INFUSION DEVICES

An alarm on the pump may be triggered by an empty bag or obstruction (e.g., infiltration, kinked tubing, air in the tubing). Alarms recognize an occlusion, air in the line, or a low battery.

- IV infusion pumps control the rate of flow and amount of solution. The pump then delivers fluid at the preset rate and amount. Different types of IV pumps can have single-channel or multichannel pumps to deliver several drugs at the same time.
- Positive-pressure infusion pumps can deliver high volumes and are used in traumas and intensive care units (ICUs).
- Volumetric pumps can deliver small volumes and are used in pediatric and neonatal settings.
- Syringe pumps are used to deliver antibiotics, patient-controlled analgesia (PCA) and drugs that are to be infused in small-volume amounts. (These pumps are limited to deliver a volume that is the size of the syringe.)
- Ambulatory pumps are used for home care patients and can be used for parenteral nutrition, pain medication, and other programmable drug schedules. They weigh less than 6 lbs and may have a backpack option for portability.
- Smart pumps are infusion pumps with dosage calculation software and are recommended to reduce adverse drug events. They may have a wireless network connection. Dose-track technology and dose-guard technology are new technologies that provide safeguards for the patient receiving the medication.
- PCA pumps can be used as epidural, continuous, or patient-controlled delivery in which the client pushes a button attached to the pump to control the administration of medication.
- IV infusion pumps require close nursing observation for early signs of infiltration and to evaluate the rate of fluid infusion and the client's response.

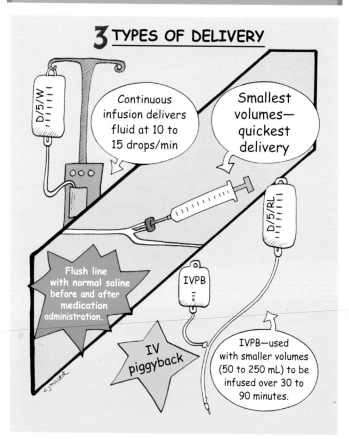

Types of Intravenous Delivery

CONTINUOUS INFUSION

Continuous infusion is used primarily for administering IV fluids.

> ***Example:*** D_5 ½ NS at 100 mL/hr

Nursing Management: Take Action

- Monitor the IV insertion site.
- Watch for infiltration (e.g., coolness with pain, swelling, tenderness at site) and phlebitis (e.g., pain, warmth, red streaks up the arm from the site).
- Use a lumen that is large enough to deliver the volume of fluid ordered for continuous infusions. Use a 20- to 22-gauge peripheral IV catheter to deliver maintenance replacement fluids. Consider using a peripherally inserted central catheter (PICC) or a central line catheter in an emergency or when IV therapy is administered for a prolonged period. When large amounts of fluid or when blood needs to be infused, use an 18-gauge catheter to allow for rapid infusion.

IV BOLUS

IV bolus is used to deliver a drug quickly (e.g., emergency or code situations) or for a fast response when needed for pain control.

> ***Example:*** Fentanyl, 25 mcg IV bolus every 30 to 60 min as needed for pain (adult opioid naïve)

Nursing Management: Take Action

- Flush the line before and after the delivery of the drug.
- Check compatibility of the drug with what is already infusing in the line.
- Instruct the client to report any of the following symptoms: redness, warmth, or numbness or pain at the IV insertion site.

INTERMITTENT INFUSION

IV piggyback (IVPB) is commonly used when administering an antibiotic or electrolyte replacement; typically used with an infusion pump.

Nursing Management: Take Action

- If using an IVPB, set up a secondary line. Hang the IVPB container at a level higher than the maintenance infusion.
- Change the IV tubing at least every 72 hours for all IV fluids and drugs.

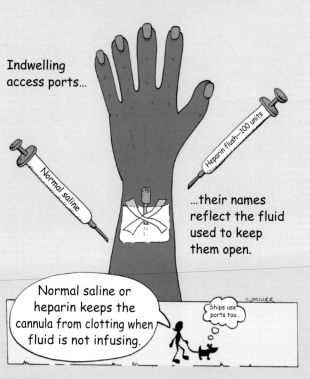

What You Need to Know
Use of Saline Locks

SALINE LOCKS

Saline locks are used to prevent an IV insertion site from clotting when IV fluids are not infusing.

Nursing Management: Take Action

- Check the institution policy and verify the type of line in place.
- Check patency of the line and lock by flushing it with 1 to 3 mL NS.
- Assess patency and blood return by gently withdrawing on the syringe.
- On flushing, check the area distal to catheter end for discomfort or swelling.
- Administer medication.
- Flush the line again with 1 to 5 mL NS, depending on institutional guidelines.

HEPARIN LOCKS

Heparin locks are used to prevent an IV insertion site from clotting when it is not being used.

Nursing Management: Take Action

- Remember the SASH method:
    - **S**aline—Flush lock with 1 mL NS.
    - **A**dminister medication.
    - **S**aline flush again to clear lock.
    - **H**eparinize with heparin flush solution.
- Check institution guidelines for heparin lock maintenance. Note the amount and concentration of heparin used to flush and maintain the line. If the line requires several milliliters to flush and flushing is frequently performed over a 24-hour period, the client can receive a significant amount of heparin. Heparin flush solutions come in the following strengths: 10 units/mL and 100 units/mL.

EXAMPLES

- Dialysis catheter
- Central line IV catheters
- Peripherally inserted central catheter (PICC)
- Butterfly catheters
- Peripheral IV catheter
- Implanted ports

COMPLICATIONS OF PERIPHERAL IV THERAPY

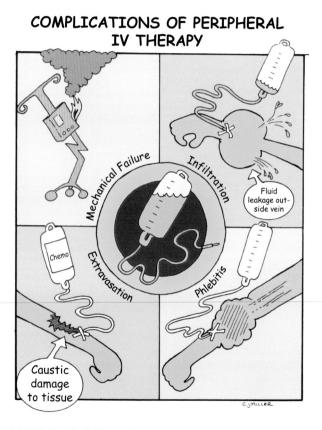

=== **What You Need to Know** ===

Complications of Peripheral Intravenous Therapy

INFILTRATION

Infiltration is caused by infusion of IV fluid or medication into surrounding tissue.

Assessment: Recognize Cues

- IV stops infusing or is significantly slower.
- Coolness of skin, pain, and tenderness surrounds the site.
- Tissue induration and swelling of tissue occurs at end of the IV catheter.
- Blood return is absent when line is drawn back, or fluid container is lowered.

Nursing Management: Take Action

- Frequently assess and document the IV site.
- Encourage the client to report signs of swelling or pain.
- Remove the catheter if infiltration is documented.
- Apply warm compresses to the infiltrated site and elevate the site.

INFILTRATION OR EXTRAVASATION OF CAUSTIC FLUIDS

Infiltration or extravasation of vesicant (caustic) fluids is most commonly caused by a medication that causes tissue necrosis in the area of infiltration.

Assessment: Recognize Cues

Burning, pain at the site, inflammation; blisters, sloughing of skin; blanching of skin

Nursing Management: Take Action

- Check institution policy regarding the removal of an IV catheter. IV antidote may be administered via the present catheter, or the catheter may be removed.
- Stop the IV infusion; apply cool compresses initially and then warm, moist compresses; elevate the site. Photograph infusion site.

PHLEBITIS

- Phlebitis is inflammation of a vein from the cannula, usually because of the length of time the cannula is in place and the infusion of irritating antibiotics or potassium.

Assessment: Recognize Cues

Redness, pain at the site, palpable cord along the vein; warmth around area

Nursing Management: Take Action

- Discontinue the IV; apply warm, moist compresses.
- All peripheral IVs should be changed every 72 to 96 hours.

CENTRAL VENOUS CATHETERS

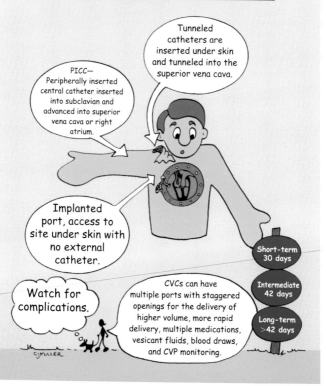

===== **What You Need to Know** =====

Central Venous Catheters

A central venous catheter (CVC) is inserted either peripherally (PICC) or directly into the subclavian; it may remain in the subclavian, or it may be progressed into the superior vena cava or right atrium.

- CVC catheters are more stable than peripheral access lines.
- Rapid access to high-volume blood flow and rapid dilution is provided when administering blood, total parenteral nutrition (TPN), chemotherapy, and emergency drugs.

TYPES OF CATHETERS

- **PICC**—A single-lumen or multilumen line is inserted peripherally into the vein slightly above the antecubital fossa and threaded through the vein into the superior vena cava. PICCs require heparinization of each lumen if the fluids are not infusing continuously. Can remain in place for months and is associated with fewer central line–associated bloodstream infections (CLABSIs).

- **Tunneled CVC**—These are inserted under the skin and tunneled into the superior vena cava. Tunneled catheters prevent skin contamination at the site of puncture from contaminating the insertion site into the vena cava and require regular heparinizations of the line when fluid is not infusing. Used for frequent and long-term infusion therapy.

- **Nontunneled CVC**—These are inserted percutaneously though the subclavian vein and exit the skin near the cannulation site. The tip of the catheter resides in the superior vena cava. Used for short-term but extensive IV therapy (e.g., multiple medications, emergent trauma situations, etc.) and are associated with a high risk of complications, including CLABSI, pneumothorax, and pulmonary embolism. Patient is placed in Trendelenburg position during insertion.

- **Implantable ports**—These are tunneled into place, and a portal or access chamber is sutured under the skin. Implantable ports may be used for months to years. The port is accessed by puncturing the skin over the port with a Huber needle. Prior to drug administration, check for a blood return. No external catheter or dressing is required over area when the catheter is not in use. Port is flushed with heparin (10 units/mL) after each use and at least once a month.

Note: Always use 10-mL syringes to flush the line, because a smaller syringe exerts pressure that could rupture the catheter.

Important nursing implications

Serious/life-threatening implications

Most frequent side effects

Patient teaching

IV Therapy

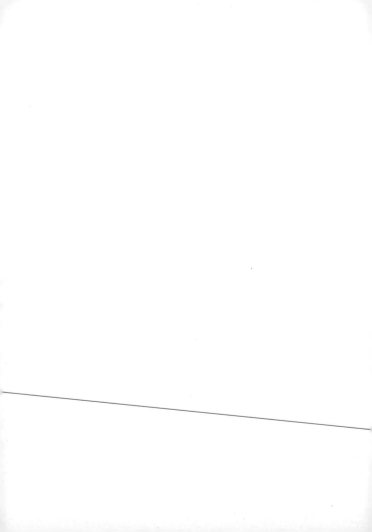

PEDIATRIC IV THERAPY

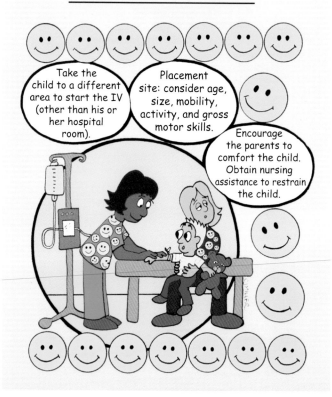

What You Need to Know
Pediatric Intravenous Therapy

Parents or caregivers should be prepared before the procedure, including an explanation of what is going to be done and the purpose of the IV fluids or catheter.

D_5W should be used with caution in children. It is rapidly metabolized, leaving free water that will increase movement of fluid into the cells, which can result in cerebral edema. NS or LR solution is frequently used for hydration.

If IV therapy is needed for more than 6 days, a midline catheter or PICC is recommended.

BEFORE THE PROCEDURE
- Preferably, take the child to the treatment room for the procedure.
- Do not ask the parents to help restrain the child during or after the procedure.
- Encourage the parents to comfort the child or infant during and after completion.
- Explain the procedure to the child based on developmental level.

EQUIPMENT
- Infusion pump should be used to regulate fluid infusion. Syringe pumps are often used because they can precisely deliver small volumes of medication.
- Use microdrip tubing (60 drops/min) to administer a small amount of fluid or medication. Equipment is designed to prevent accidental bolus infusion.

NURSING IMPLICATIONS: TAKE ACTION
- Monitor fluid balance (intake and output [I&O], daily weights), vital signs.
- Add supplemental potassium to IV fluids only after the child has voided and kidney function has been validated.
- Follow the same guidelines as used for adults when selecting the site.
- Wrap the extremity in a warm pack to increase vasodilation and visibility of the vein prior to insertion of a short-term peripheral IV.
- Use a small tourniquet or blood pressure cuff.
- Do not attempt to start an IV on a child or infant alone; obtain assistance in restraining.
- Do not tape or wrap all the way around the extremity; doing so can cause obstruction if swelling occurs.

Important nursing implications	Serious/life-threatening implications
Most frequent side effects	Patient teaching

Index

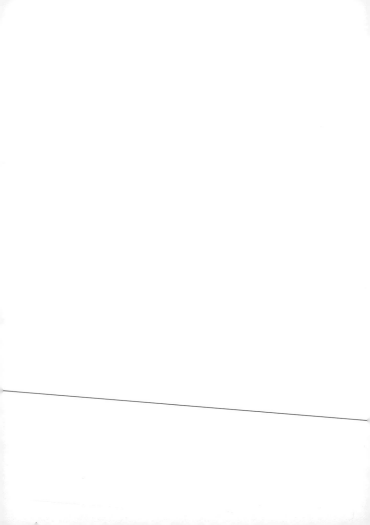